LEPROSY
IN FIVE YOUNG MEN

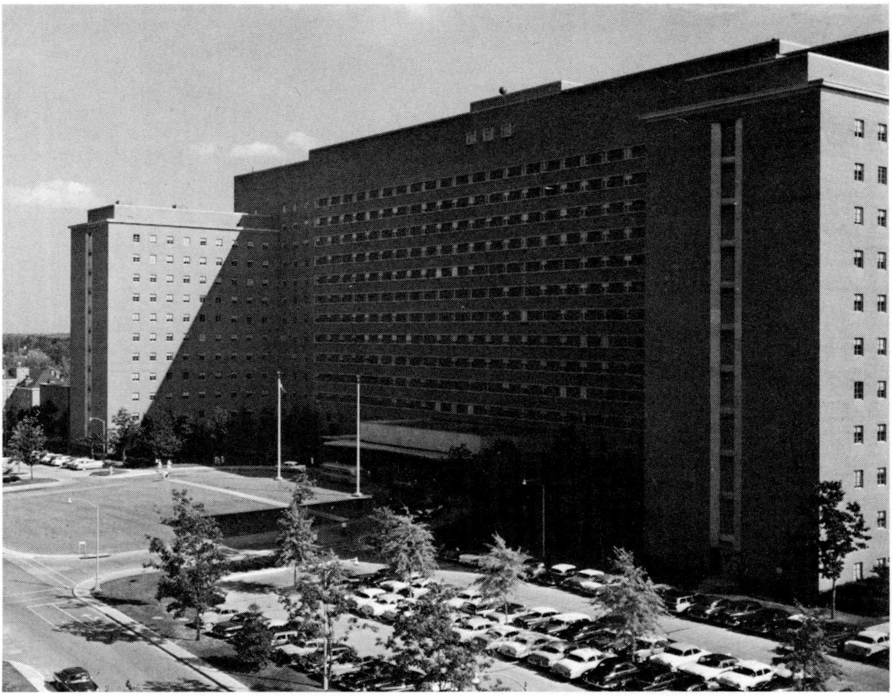

Fig. 1. Clinical Center, National Institutes of Health, Bethesda, Md.

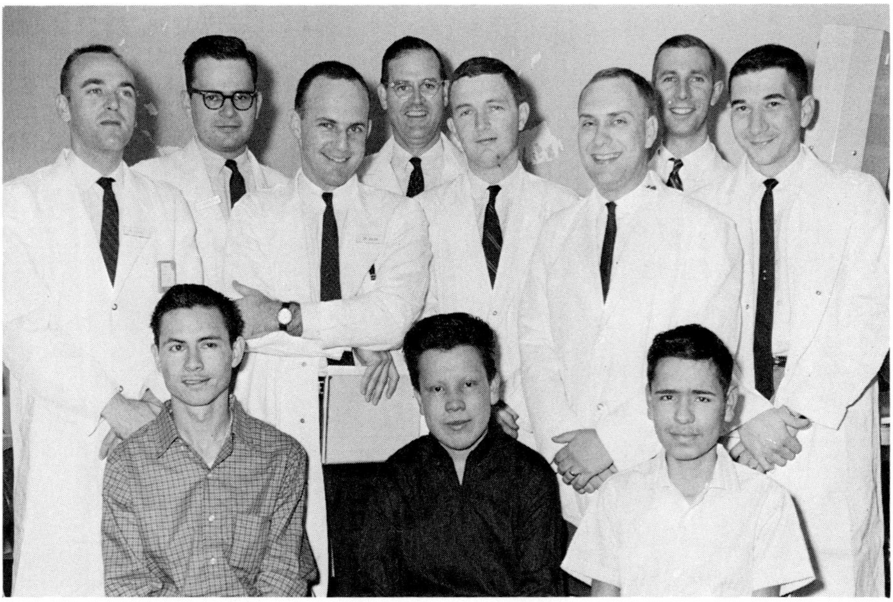

Fig. 2. Clinical Center staff and patients. Patients, *front row, left to right,* 2, 1 and 3. Physicians, *left to right,* Drs. Benjamin Sturgill, Melvin Rubenstein, Richard Adler, Vernon Knight, John Mulholland, James Smith, George Hill, and William Fleet.

LEPROSY

IN FIVE YOUNG MEN

George J. Hill, II, M.D., F.A.C.S.

Assistant Professor of Surgery
University of Colorado School of Medicine
Denver, Colorado

formerly Clinical Associate
National Institutes of Health
Bethesda, Maryland

COLORADO ASSOCIATED UNIVERSITY PRESS

1970

Colorado Associated University Press
1424 Fifteenth Street
Boulder, Colorado 80302

Library of Congress Catalog Card Number 79–125621
ISBN 87081–003–0

TO

E. M. H.

CONTENTS

ILLUSTRATIONS

PATIENT 3

PATIENT 4

TABLES

PREFACE

This work was initiated by the imaginative effort of Dr. Vernon Knight, as clinical director of the National Institute of Allergy and Infectious Diseases (NIAID). The collaborative international effort derived enthusiastic support from our colleagues in Mexico, principally Dr. Fernando Latapí and Dr. José Barba Rubio.*

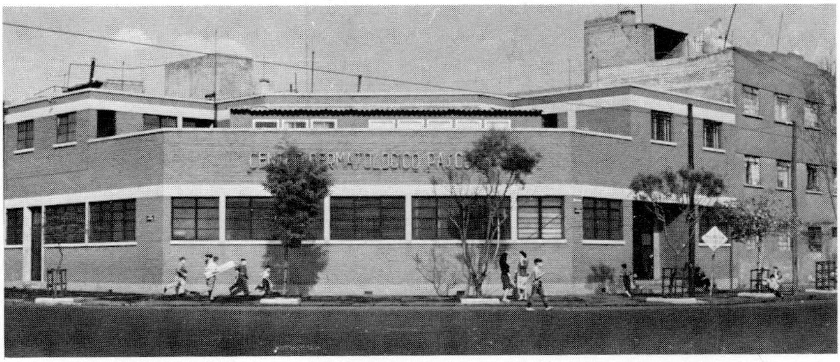

Fig. 3. Centra Dermatologico Pascua, Mexico City, Mexico.

The decision to bring aliens with untreated leprosy to Bethesda, Maryland, was the contribution of many men, in particular Dr. C. K. Himmelsbach, associate director of the Clinical Center, National Institutes of Health (NIH), and Dr. Dorland Davis, scientific director, NIAID. Careful thought was given to the project before it was approved by the NIH and the Department of Health, Education and Welfare. Cooperation was given by the Immigration and Naturalization Service, the Department of State, and Department of Justice in the United States. Valuable assistance was also given by the Embassy of Mexico, Mexican Ministry of Health (Secretaria de Salubridad y Asistencia), the governor of Jalisco, and Brig. Gen. Paredes Menchaca, Jefe Estado Mayor, Mexico City.

The project was carried out in collaboration with the Leonard Wood Memorial, through the assistance of its medical director,

* Dr. Latapí is director of the Centro Dermatologico Pascua, Dr. Garcia Diego 21, Colonia Doctores, Mexico, 7, D.F., Mexico (associate director, Dr. Amado Sául). Dr. Barba Rubio is director of the Instituto Dermatologico Guadalajara, Avenida Independence 66, Guadalajara, Mexico (associate director, Dr. Gloria Pérez Suárez).

the late Dr. James A. Doull, and Dr. John Hanks and Dr. Chapman Binford. Participating organizations in Mexico included the Asociación Mexicana de Acción contra la Lepra, Dermatologia Revista Mexicana, Organizado por la Soc. Mexicana de Dermatologia, the Centro Dermatologico Pascua, and the Instituto Dermatologico, Guadalajara. Dr. Amado Saúl and Dr. Gloria Pérez Suárez were particularly helpful in this work. Sra. Latapí and Sra. Barba Rubio were especially kind to us and to the young men with leprosy.

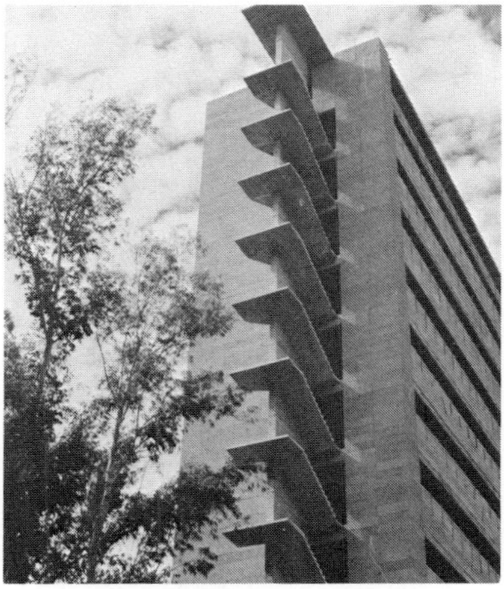

Fig. 4. A wing of Hospital General, Guadalajara, Jalisco, Mexico. Here are hospitalized patients of Instituto Dermatologico Guadalajara.

The investigations were carried out with the aid of many other members of the staff at the NIH Clinical Center. Dr. Richard Adler was my associate during the period when the clinical studies were performed, 1962–63, and the text was reviewed by Drs. John Singleton and William Butler. The initial uncertainty and trembling on the part of the clinical staff was overcome, in good measure, by the calm encouragement of Mrs. Betty Kuster, administrative assistant for the Laboratory of Clinical Investigation. The manuscript was reviewed by the NIAID, and permission for its publication was given on 1 October 1969 by Dr. Sheldon Wolff, clinical director. Dr. Wolff also made the valuable suggestion that terminology of the immunoglobulins be changed to the current usage, rather than the form used in 1962–63. I have endeavored to incorporate the recommendations of the reviewers, which are hereby gratefully acknowledged. This book is not an official publication of the U.S. Public Health Service (USPHS), and the opinions expressed are solely those of the author.

The advice and assistance given by others in the scientific community was most welcome. The late Dr. Edgar Johnwick, medical director of the USPHS Hospital, Carville, La., offered his hospitality and guidance to us in the early months of the study, when support was greatly needed. We were also grateful for suggestions made by Dr. George L. Fite, Dr. R. J. W. Rees, and Dr. Charles Shepard.

The voluntary participation of the five young patients was essential to the success of the study. The patients and their parents were fully cooperative in all respects, and I am grateful for their permission to perform the studies and to publish the results.

Permission to quote passages in published works is acknowledged. The Clarendon Press, Oxford, kindly granted permission to quote from "The Testament of Cresseid' by Robert Henryson, a modernized excerpt from *Chaucerian and Other Pieces,* Vol. 7, ed. Walter W. Skeat (1897). Permission to quote from Robert Louis Stevenson's poem "To Mother Maryanne" was given by Charles Scribner's Sons, publishers of *The Complete Poems of Robert Louis Stevenson* (1905). The publisher's permission was given to quote excerpts from *Damien the Leper* by John Farrow, Sheed & Ward (1st ed., 1937), and from S. V. Larkey, a note on "Testament of Cresseid," *Bull. Hist. Med.* 35:77 (1961). The quotation from Betty Martin, *No One Must Ever Know,* is used with permission of Doubleday and Co. (1959). Permission to quote from Perry Burgess, *Who Walk Alone,* was given by the publisher, Holt, Rinehart and Winston, New York. Figure 1 is published with the consent of Brooks Photographers, Bethesda, Maryland.

My deepest gratitude goes to my wife for her encouragement to continue the preparation of this report until it was complete. The final drafts of this monograph were prepared during the tenure of a Lederle Medical Faculty Award, and this assistance was greatly appreciated.

George J. Hill II, M.D., F.A.C.S.
Denver, January 20, 1970

INTRODUCTION

"To see the infinite pity of this place,
The mangled limb, the devastated face,
The innocent sufferers smiling at the rod,
A fool were tempted to deny his God."

Robert Louis Stevenson
writing about the Molokai Leprosy Colony, Hawaii.

Leprosy is the greatest paradox of infectious diseases. Although it was one of the first diseases discovered to be related to microorganisms, it is still an enigma, because the causative organism is exceedingly difficult to propagate and transmit. The mystery of leprosy is compounded by a long incubation period, the difficulty of early diagnosis, and — above all — by ignorance and fear. In addition, leprosy is more resistant to chemotherapy than is any other bacterial disease.

Each of the problems in leprosy is an important challenge, for the movement of the world's growing population results in increasing contact between susceptible travelers and the 12 million patients* who have leprosy. Today's means of rapid transportation make it possible for patients with leprosy to travel in countries where this disease is rare, and where resistance may be low.

In order to determine what new research programs might be undertaken in leprosy, NIAID began a new clinical study of leprosy in 1962. This study was carried out at the NIH Clinical Center (Figs. 1, 2) in Bethesda, Maryland, under the auspices of the U.S. Public Health Service and the Department of Health, Education, and Welfare. The major goal of the study was to stimulate the interest of medical and biological scientists in diverse fields, who might thereby make original contributions to the solution of the problem of leprosy. It seemed appropriate to organize the research efforts around specific questions concerning individual patients.

* New York Academy of Sciences, 1966.

The first objective of the study was to describe the abnormalities which the patients presented. The findings are presented in this monograph.

It was considered desirable to study young patients who were still in the early phases of their disease, and who had not received therapy. A source of young untreated patients, upon whom epidemiological and followup studies could easily be arranged, was made available through a cooperative program with two large clinics in Mexico, the Centro Dermatologico Pascua, Mexico City (Fig. 3) and the Instituto Dermatologico, Guadalajara (Fig. 4). The first patients were admitted to the Clinical Center in May 1962; over the next year a total of five patients were admitted for study. The period of observation and medical tests for each patient lasted two to three months. This period is designated in each case as Study Period I. In four patients the initial observation period was followed by a period of therapy designated Study Period II. Comparative observations were repeated during periods of therapy which ranged from three to seven months.

None of these five young men had previously been hospitalized, and none was totally disabled by leprosy. Two were working at their usual occupations, and three were living quietly at home when they were selected to come to the United States. One patient was unaware that he had any disease; he was discovered only as a result of epidemiologic studies of his mother, who was symptomatic with lepromatous leprosy. Nevertheless, the five patients showed extensive pathologic changes. Many, but not all, of the abnormalities were due to infection with leprosy. It is the purpose of this report to describe and classify these abnormalities. Some of the lesions will be shown to be the result of bacterial invasion and adjacent inflammation, whereas other abnormalities are due to therapy or intercurrent diseases.

METHODS

> "We have suffered too long in loneliness and fear . . . We belong with the secret people . . . We are always afraid."
>
> Betty Martin
> *No One Must Ever Know*

The five patients in this study were selected from a group of approximately 8,000 outpatients with leprosy who are treated at the Centro Dermatologico Pascua, Mexico City, and the Instituto Dermatologico, Guadalajara, Mexico. It was customary for all patients admitted to the clinics to be interviewed by physicians and social workers. Normal intelligence and a spirit of cooperation were looked for in potential candidates for the study. The five who were selected were among recent admissions to the clinics, were under 30 years of age, and had received no prior therapy for leprosy. The disease had first been diagnosed in each of them only one to two months previously.

The patients were initially chosen as representative examples of "types" of leprosy. However, in some cases the lack of stability in the clinical course led to difficulty in making a definite assessment of classification. In each case the diagnosis of leprosy was established on the basis of non-cultivable acid-fast bacilli in his cutaneous or nasal tissues, and by demonstration of anesthesia in some area of the body.

All five of the patients selected for observation and therapy were males. Because of social and psychological problems associated with bringing young women to the United States, only males were considered as candidates. The young men had in common their national origin (Mexico), race (mestizo, a mixture of Caucasian and American Indian), birth and residence in leprosy endemic areas (the states of Jalisco, Nayarit, Michoacan, and the Federal District), and the common denominator of extreme poverty.

While similarities in the patients have been emphasized, it should be mentioned that the patients differed grossly in the manifestations of leprosy which they presented. They came from somewhat dissimilar urban or rural backgrounds (three were born on farms and two in large cities). For this reason they represented dissimilar social environments with accompanying differences in diet.

The length of exposure in each case to persons known to have leprosy also was a variable. Members of the immediate families of three of the patients had leprosy, but the index cases for the other two patients were unknown. While the patients had their youth in common, they represented a wide range of personal development; one had recently reached puberty, one was a married father, and two of the others (in their twenties) had experienced extensive extra-marital sexual activity.

The studies performed on each of the patients were similar in many respects; the patients had in common a prolonged continuous hospitalization prior to and during therapy. Hospitalization made it possible to control diet and environment, to perform frequent measurements of weight and height, to collect specimens, and to manage therapy with optimum accuracy and safety.

Since many of the investigations required techniques which were available only on a research basis, studies were performed in collaboration with consultants from different laboratories at the Clinical Center. The technical details of the tests made are described in this monograph under the appropriate sections of the Discussion, which is divided into twelve parts corresponding to the twelve systems studied. The research studies performed, and the consultants who performed them, are listed in Table 1.

Although a general similarity was present in the studies of the five patients, some differences did exist. For example, since the erythema nodosum reactions in two patients occasionally interfered with their planned programs, the period prior to therapy in those cases varied from two to three and a half months. Four of the five patients were observed, during the initial phase of their therapy, for periods lasting from three to seven months. The therapeutic regimens followed in these patients were also somewhat variable.

All four patients received conventional therapy with 4–4′-

diaminodiphenyl sulfone (DDS).* Sulfone therapy alone was given to two patients. One of these two patients had the greatest numbers of leprosy bacilli present in his tissues prior to therapy, and the other had the least bacilli present. Sulfone therapy was also given to a third patient, who developed fever, erythema nodosum and peripheral neuropathy after three months; his therapy was then changed to diphenyl thiourea (DPT).** The fourth patient was treated simultaneously with DDS and Geigy B-663,*** a rimizine dye which has been effective against murine leprosy.

*
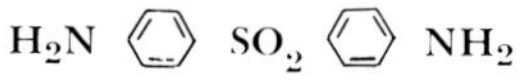

4–4′-diaminodiphenylsulfone (DDS, or Dapsone, or Avlosulfon® Ayerst)

**
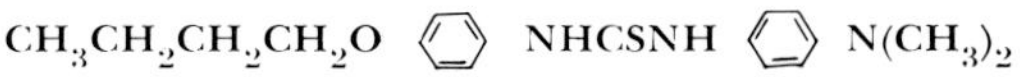

4,butoxy-4′, dimethylaminodiphenyl thiourea
(thiocarbanilide, or CIBA 1906, or DPT)

***
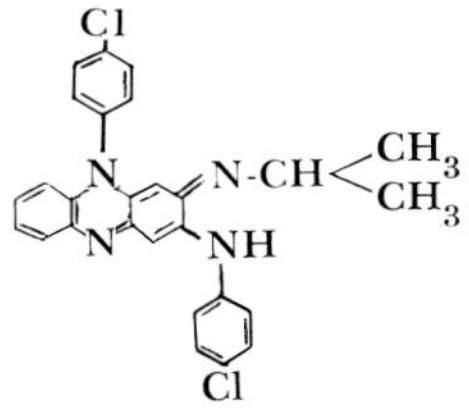

Geigy B-663

CASE SUMMARIES

"Unless this place is to become another Devil's Island where hope is surrendered at entrance, belief in return must remain with us."

Perry Burgess, *Who Walk Alone*

PATIENT 1

A 17-Year Old Male of Mestizo Extraction

Leprosy caused extensive tissue destruction, pancytopenia and aspermatogenesis (Figs. 5 and 6). Tentative Diagnosis: Lepromatous leprosy, diffuse, with Lucio phenomenon. Final Diagnosis: Same.

History. Slowly healing, painful ulcerations of the legs (Fig. 7) had been present for six years. The patient had been kept out of school because of these lesions, which his mother believed were "contagious." He noticed paresthesias of the extremities and muscular weakness in his hands shortly after the lesions first appeared on his legs. Rhinitis, recurrent epistaxis, and alopecia of the eyebrows and eyelashes had first been observed four years prior to admission, and had become progressively more severe. He had noticed the gradual development of malaise, weakness and anorexia, but he was unaware of any acute illnesses or fevers.

The patient had been treated unsuccessfully with vitamins and antibiotics for his generalized debilitation. The diagnosis of leprosy had been made only one month prior to admission, when he was taken to the Centro Dermatologico Pascua for treatment of the leg lesions. These lesions had the characteristic dark surface, angular margins and underlying thrombotic lepromatous arteritis characteristic of the Lucio phenomenon.

Epidemiological Data. The patient's birth place and home is in a rural suburban area in the southeastern part of Mexico City, known as the Ixtacalco sector, 3.5 miles southeast of Mexico City's cathedral and 6 miles northeast of the University of Mexico. The population of Mexico City is rapidly increasing; it totalled approximately 4.6 million in 1962. Mexico City has a temperate climate because of its high altitude (7,300 feet), although it lies 4° south of the Tropic of Cancer.

Nothing is known about the patient's father, and his present family group consists of his grandmother, his mother and stepfather, five half-siblings, and fourteen aunts, uncles and cousins, all of whom live together in a cluster of five rooms which surround a small courtyard (Fig. 8). The dwellings have electricity but no running water. Chickens and other domestic animals wander freely through the rooms. An outdoor privy is used for waste disposal, and there is no septic tank. The compound is crowded, but it is clean and free from offensive odors. The family is apparently happy and in generally good health. The children sleep upon rugs on the dirt floors of the rooms, and the infants and adults sleep in beds. Only the patient and his grandmother have single beds.

Between the ages of one and three the patient had slept in the same bed with his grandfather, who is now dead. His grandfather is said to have had "sores" on his legs similar to those which the patient now has. The only other person in his family who is known to have leprosy is his three year old half-sister, who was discovered by an epidemiologic survey to have a tuberculoid leprosy macule of the right eyebrow (Fig. 9).

Hospitalization at the Clinical Center (Fig. 10). In Study Period I, which lasted for two months, the patient's course was remarkably stable, as measured by clinical and laboratory examinations. He developed new leg lesions at a relatively constant rate (six in the two-month period). His weight increased 2.5 kg, to 47 kg. He exhibited paresis and anesthesia of a small area in the distribution of the right ulnar nerve (Fig. 13). Leprosy bacilli and globi were demonstrated in his skin, lymph nodes, bone marrow, blood (Fig. 25), liver, testicles, testicular fasciae, subcutaneous tissue, sputum, gastric washings and semen. Acid fast bacilli were also found in kidney, perirenal fat, gum, jejunem, prostate and hydrocele fluid.

The patient initially demonstrated a subnormal response to ACTH, and exhibited testicular atrophy, pancytopenia, reticulocytosis, hepatosplenomegaly, hyperglobulinemia and multiple nonspecific positive serological reactions. He had a "negative" response to intradermal lepromin. Abnormalities in x-rays (Figs. 11, 12), biopsies (Figs. 14–22) and Cr^{51} studies of red blood cell survival (Figs. 23, 24) are illustrated in accompanying figures.

Specific anti-leprosy chemotherapy was administered to the patient for the first time during Study Period II, which lasted for five months. DDS was begun at a dose of 50 mg per day for 17 days, followed by 75 mg per day for eight days, and then raised to 100 mg per day. No adverse reactions to the drug were observed, with the possible exception of an increase in circulating reticulocytes (Fig. 10 and Table 9) while he was receiving DDS.

A 50 percent shortening of the Cr^{51} red blood cell half-life was also observed at this time, but since comparable studies were not done prior to therapy it was not possible to ascribe the increased rate of red cell hemolysis to sulfone toxicity.

The patient remained free of fever and other acute reactions during his entire hospitalization. His general appearance showed little change, although he gained an additional 4.3 kg in weight. His muscular strength increased from 87 percent to 96.5 percent of normal during the five month period of DDS therapy.

During the latter part of Study Period II leprosy bacilli could no longer be recovered from the patient's sputum (Fig. 10 and Table 4), gastric washings, seminal emission or blood. His erythrocyte sedimentation rate (ESR) was generally lower than it had been on admission (Fig. 10). His serum globulin decreased gradually (Table 7) and he exhibited a more normal response to ACTH stimulation (Tables 12, 13) after receiving DDS for five months. However, skin scrapings and biopsies, a lymph node biopsy, and a bone marrow aspiration continued to show many leprosy bacilli, and his reactivity to intradermal lepromin continued to be "negative."

This young man returned to his family and his community in a remarkably improved state. He felt well, he was highly motivated, and he had improved his command of the English language. Any uneasiness which his neighbors previously felt about his illness apparently disappeared after his return. He took up life again in Mexico fully equipped to perform clerical work in a large firm. However, the great tragedy of his life was known only to him and to his physicians: because of prolonged delay in diagnosis, leprosy had rendered him a eunuch.

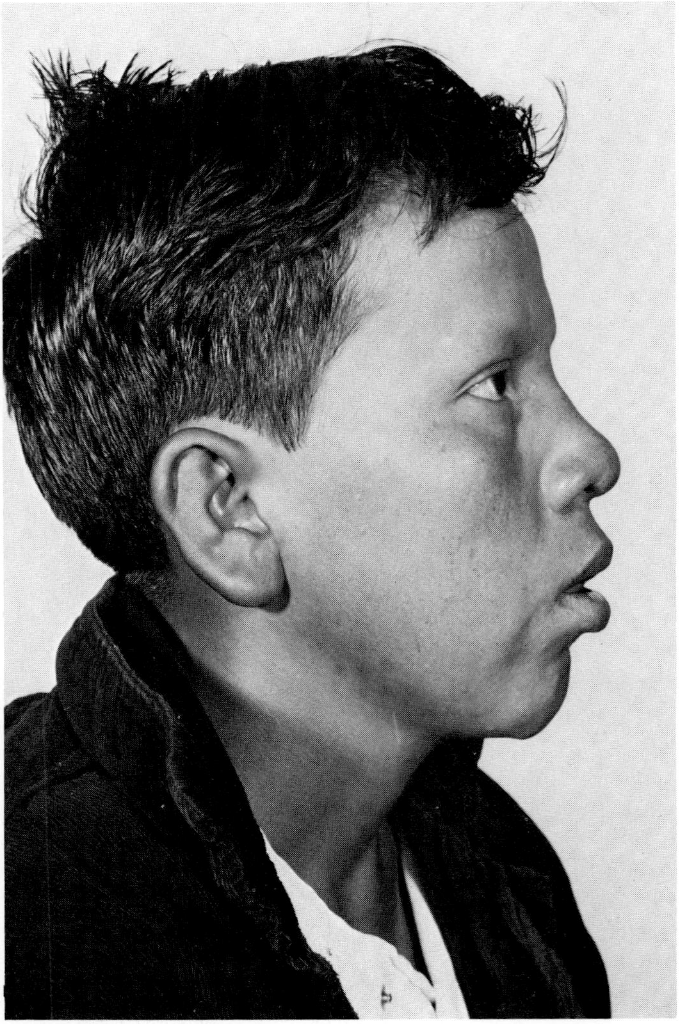

Fig. 5. Lepromatous leprosy, diffuse, in a 17-year-old male. Facial hair virtually absent; alopecia of eyebrows, edema of face, enlargement of earlobes, nasal alae, and malar eminences. Patient breathes through mouth because of severe rhinitis. (Pt. 1)

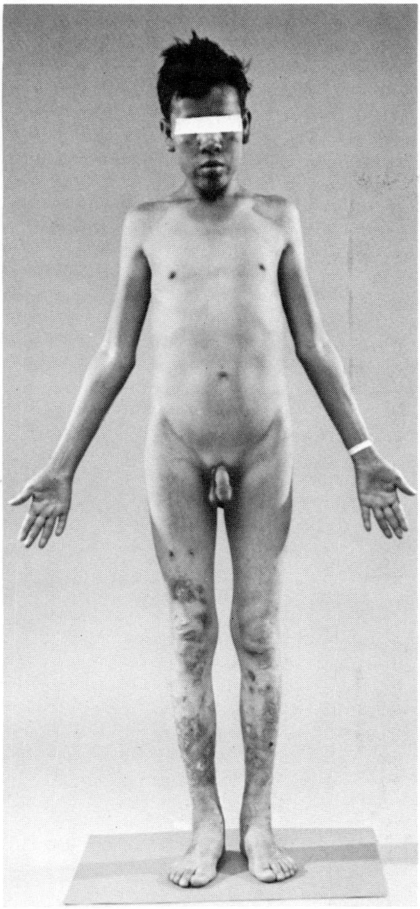

Fig. 6. Diminution of body hair, Lucio lesions of legs; testicles are small. Hands show typical features of diffuse leprosy—smooth surfaces with edema, wrinkle formation and loss of calluses. Fingers tapered, medial deviation of fifth digits.

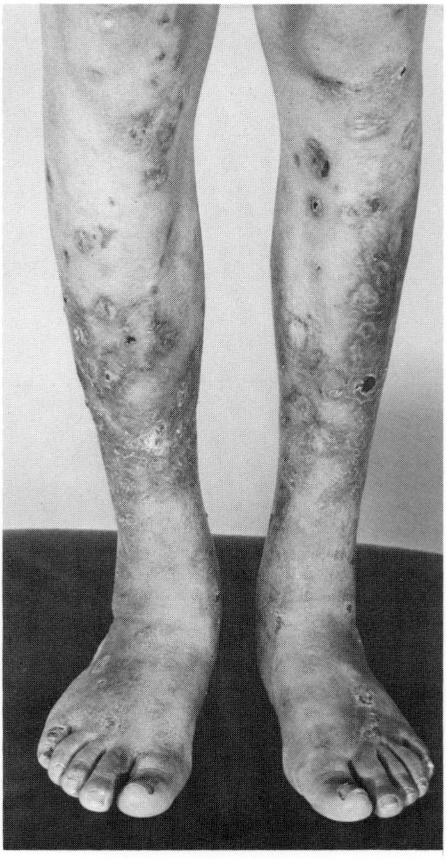

Fig. 7. Lucio lesions of legs in all stages of development and resolution. Old scars (on right patella and at left tibial tubercle) may be soft and pliable; more recent scars (on lower legs) are thick and firm. Dark lesion on left upper medial pretibial area is early hemorrhagic lesion. Other dark areas are secondary eschars over ulcerations. (Pt. 1)

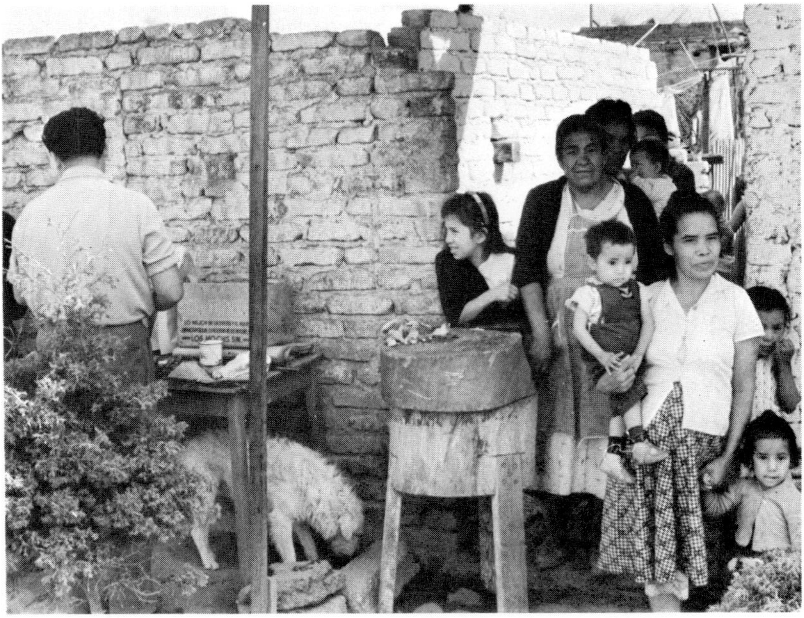

Fig. 8. Family of patient 1 at entrance to family courtyard. Low adobe brick buildings each contain two rooms. Chopping block for open-air butcher shop in center of photograph.

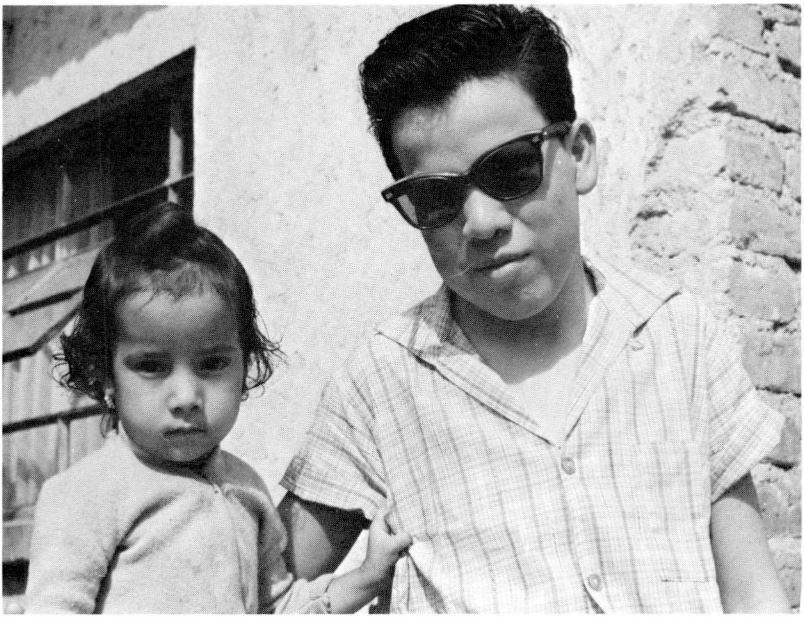

Fig. 9. Patient 1 with his three and a half-year-old half-sister, who has tuberculoid leprosy. Her raised, erythematous, anesthetic lesion of right eyebrow is only manifestation of leprosy. Lepromin skin test positive.

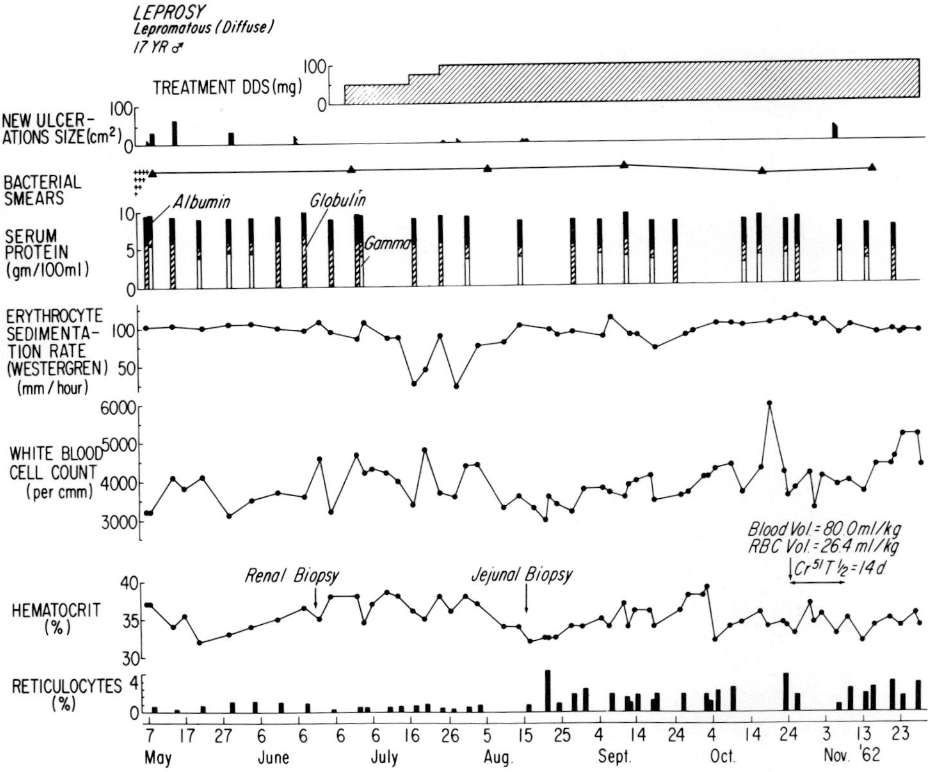

Fig. 10. Clinical Course Chart. Decreases are observed in bacterial density, serum globulin and sedimentation rate. Elevation in white blood cell count in October 1962 was caused by ACTH test. Reticulocytosis developed after six weeks of therapy. (Pt. 1)

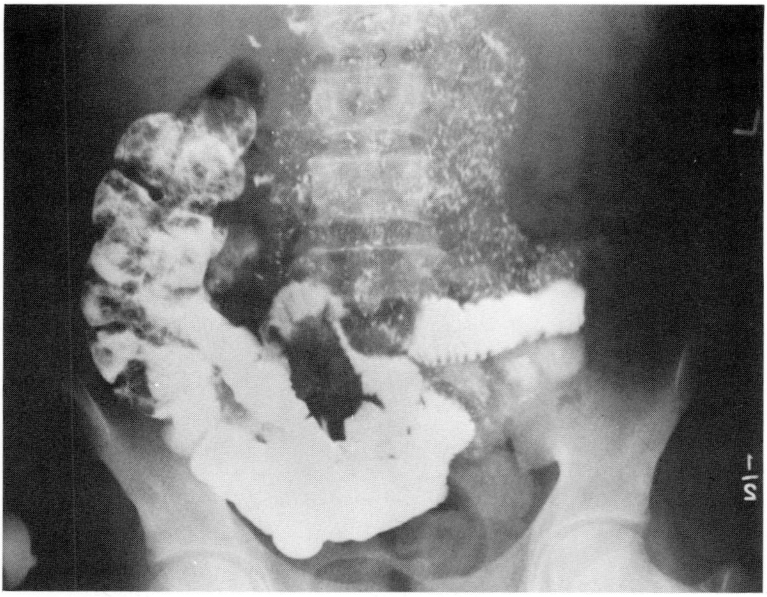

Fig. 11. X-ray, gastrointestinal series. Hepatosplenomegaly demonstrated by indentation of barium sulfate-filled small bowel by spleen, and by depression of hepatic flexure of colon by the liver. (Pt. 1)

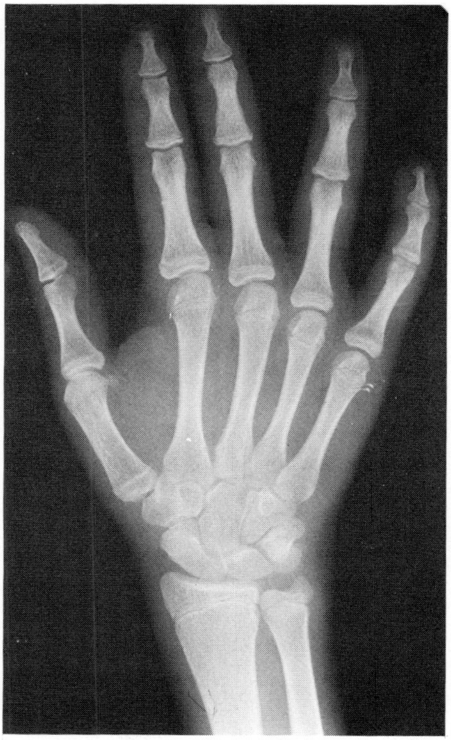

Fig. 12. X-ray, hands. Tapered phalanges in soft tissues due to destruction of dermal appendages and terminal sensory nerves. Bones are normal. (Pt. 1)

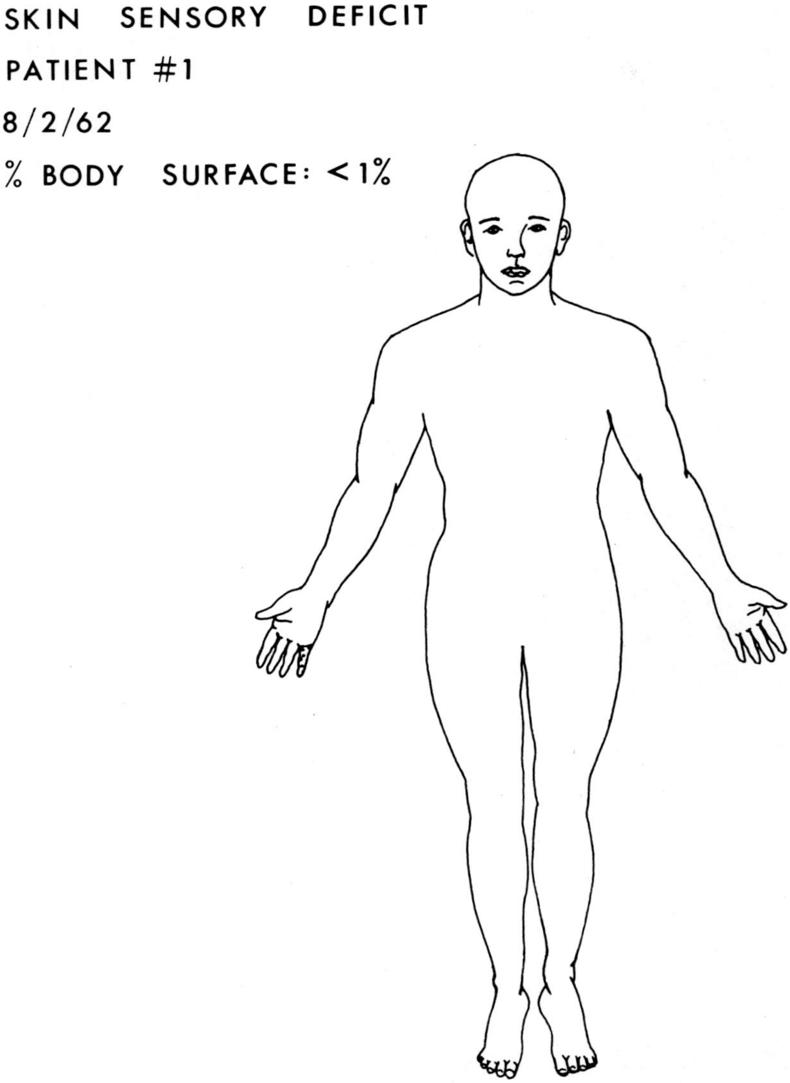

Fig. 13. Skin sensory deficit. Hypesthesia only on right fifth finger. (Pt. 1)

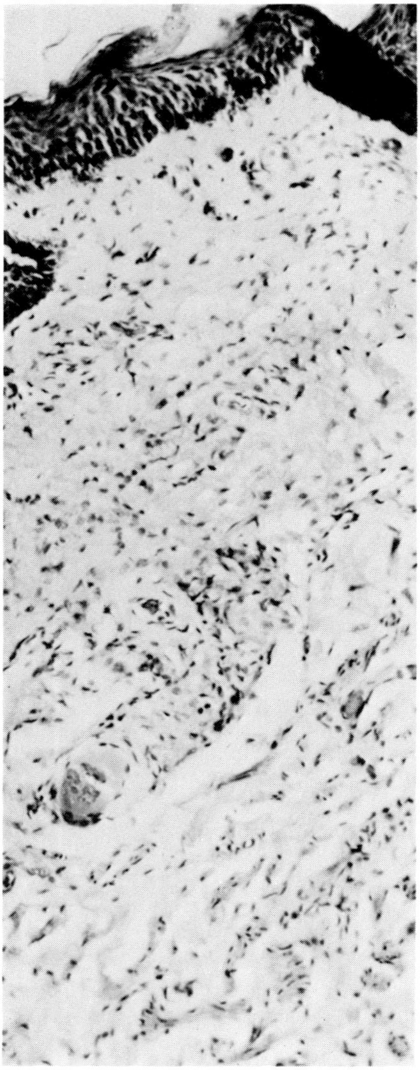

Fig. 14. Photomicrograph, scrotum. Subcutaneous inflammation and perivascular infiltration. Hematoxylin and eosin (H & E) stain, 128X (Pt. 1)

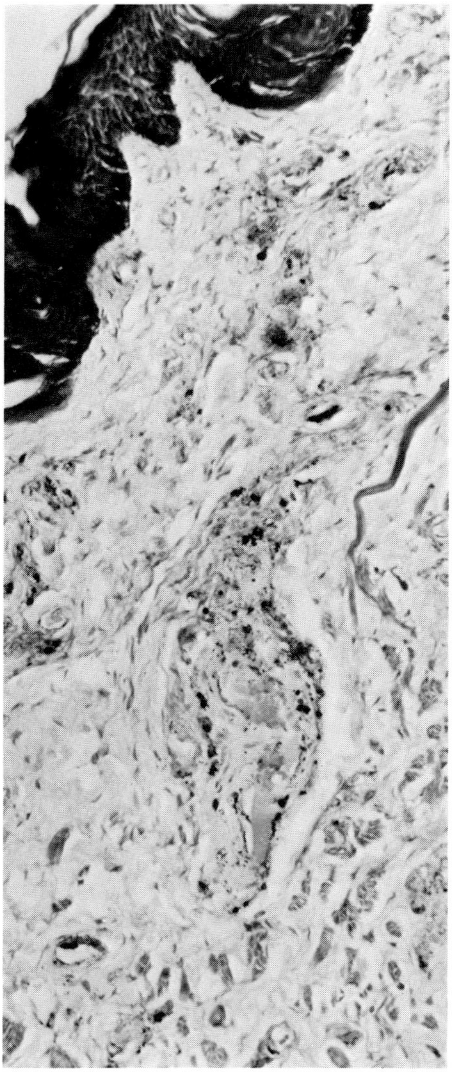

Fig. 15. Photomicrograph, scrotum. Same area as Fig. 14, cut on deeper section. Myriads of leprosy bacilli are seen here with Fite stain, 139X (Pt. 1)

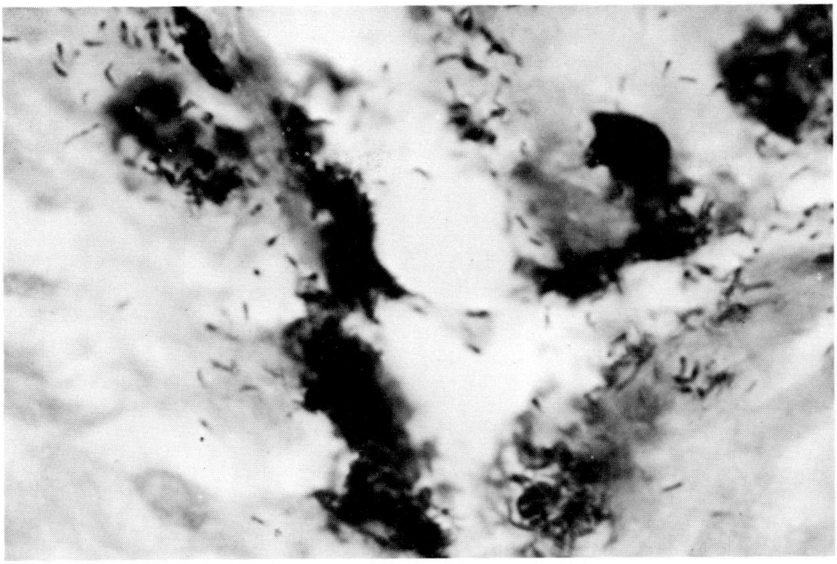

Fig. 16. Photomicrograph, abdominal wall fat. Severe lepromatous change of subcutaneous tissues is illustrated by blood vessel, either small capillary or lymphatic, with many acid-fast bacilli in its lumen, in endothelial cells, and in adjacent areas. Fite stain, 1656X. (Pt. 1)

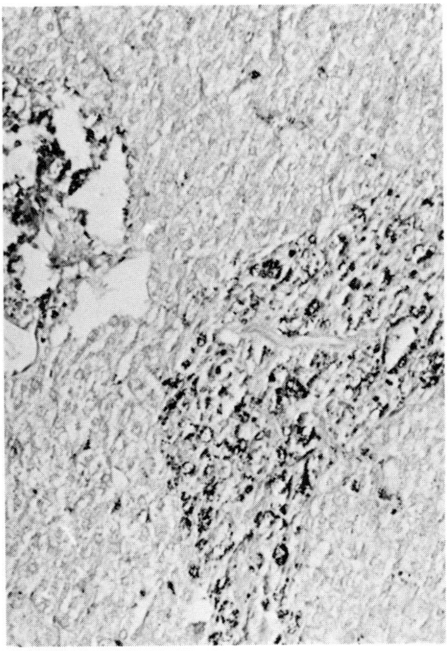

Fig. 17. Photomicrograph, liver. Necrosis in peripheral and lobular areas, with inflammatory cells and leprosy bacilli. Fite stain, 137X. (Pt. 1)

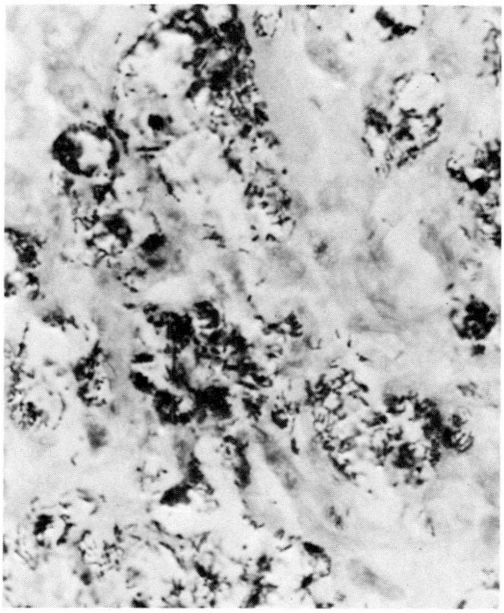

Fig. 18. Photomicrograph, liver. Masses of leprosy bacilli in large mononuclear cells (Virchow's "foam cells") and lying free in necrotic areas. Many are bipolar, club shaped, bent, angular, or curved. Fite stain, 798X. (Pt. 1)

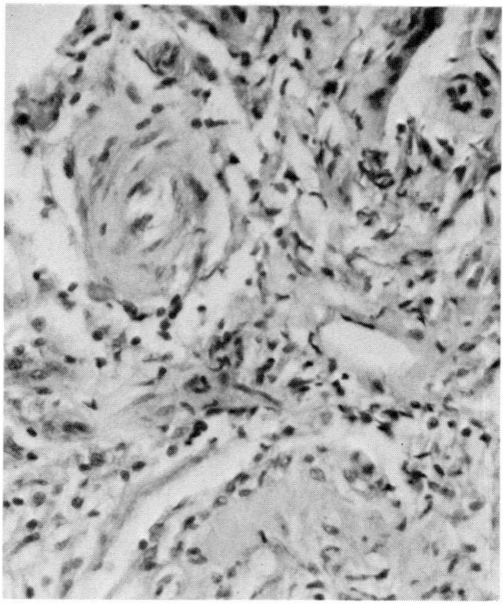

Fig. 20. Photomicrograph, testicle. Total destruction of spermatogenesis, severe inflammation, fibrosis, necrosis, and arteritis; large numbers of leprosy bacilli. H & E stain, 798X. (Pt. 1)

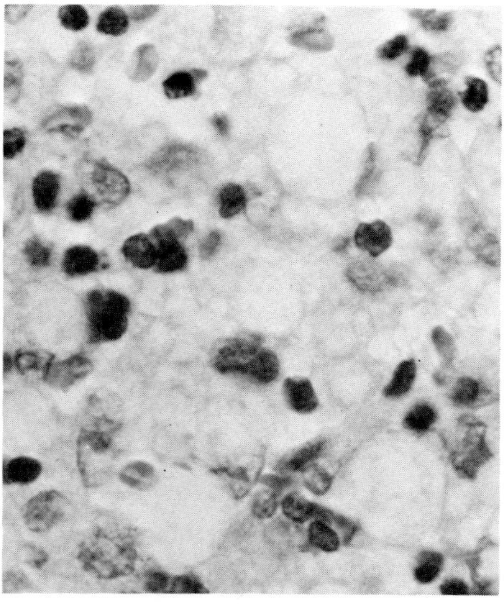

Fig. 19. Photomicrograph, lymph node. Foam cells abundant, contain masses of leprosy bacilli revealed on acid-fast stain; H & E stain, 798X. (Pt. 1)

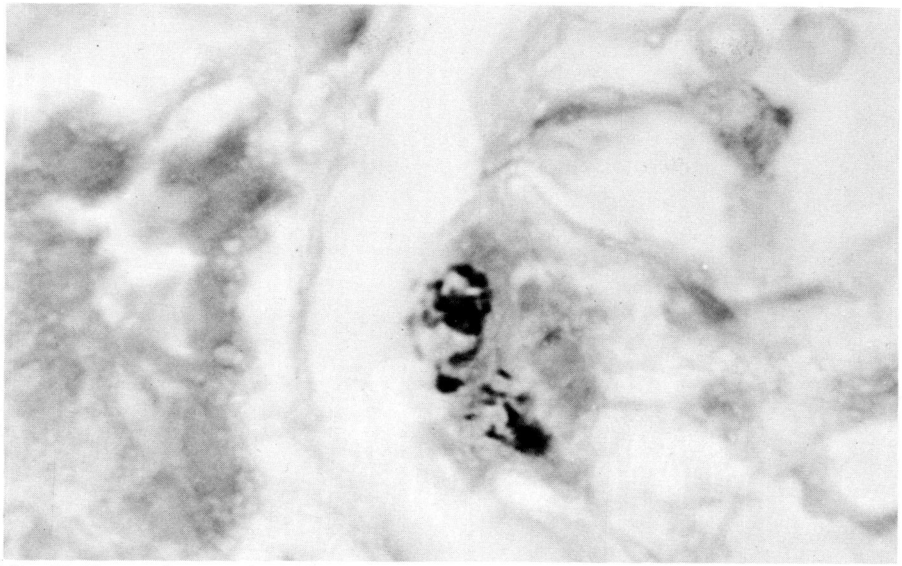

Fig. 21 Photomicrograph, kidney. Clusters of leprosy bacilli in endothelial cells of glomerulus, at basement membrane. Fite stain, 1627X. (Pt. 1)

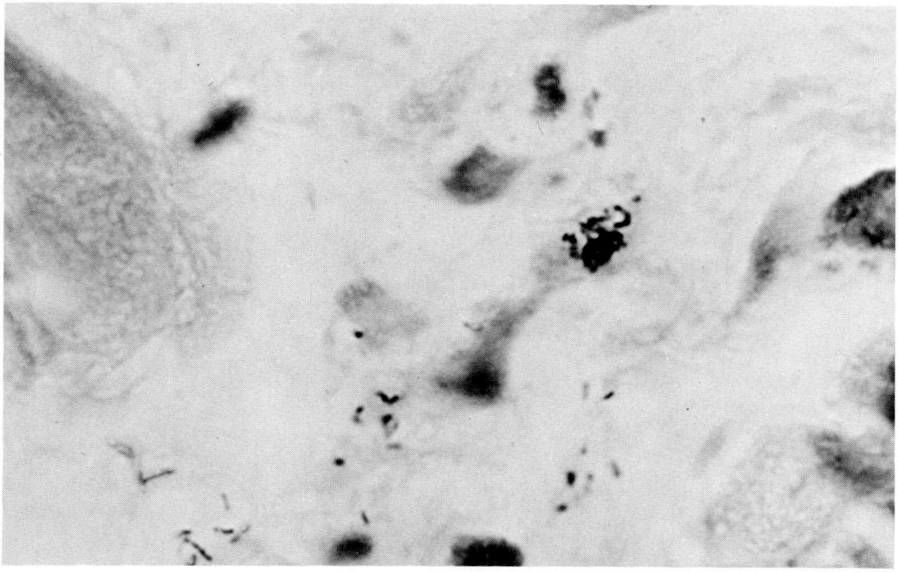

Fig. 22. Photomicrograph, prostate. Leprosy bacilli in stroma, with no associated inflammation. Fite stain, 1555X. (Pt. 1)

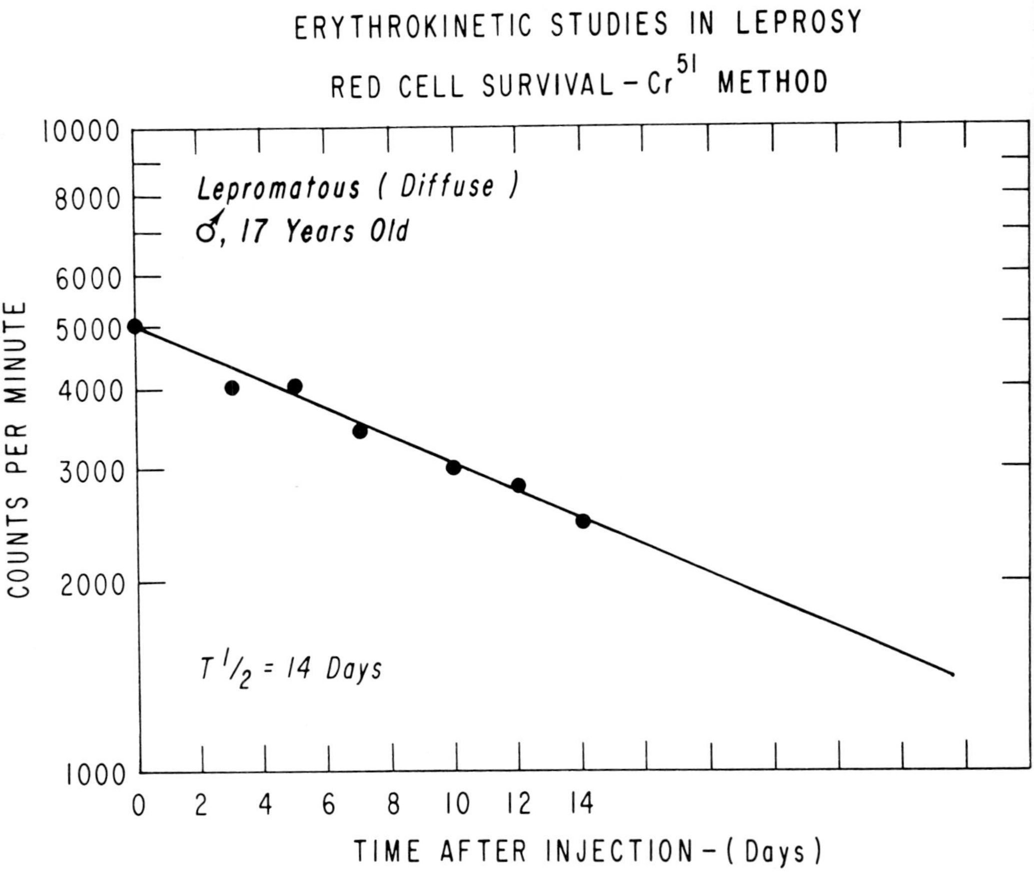

Fig. 23. Hemolytic anemia studied with Cr^{51} RBC labelling. Anemia was present prior to therapy; reticulocytosis developed after sulfones were administered. Total blood volume normal (80.0 ml/kg), although red cell mass decreased (26.4 ml/kg). (Pt. 1)

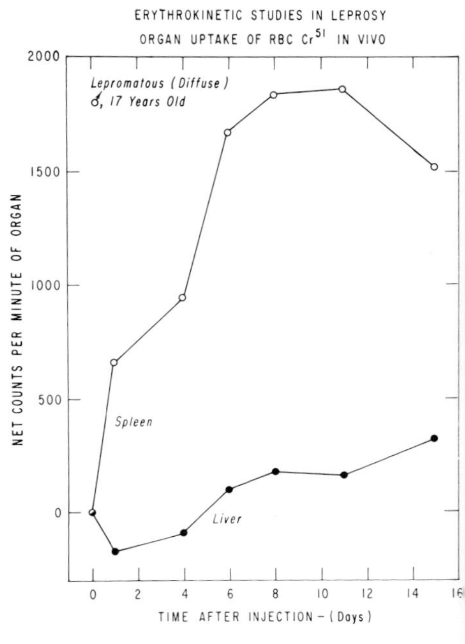

Fig. 24. Splenic red cell trapping demonstrated by surface measurement of radioactivity with Geiger counter after RBC labelling with Cr^{51}. (Pt. 1)

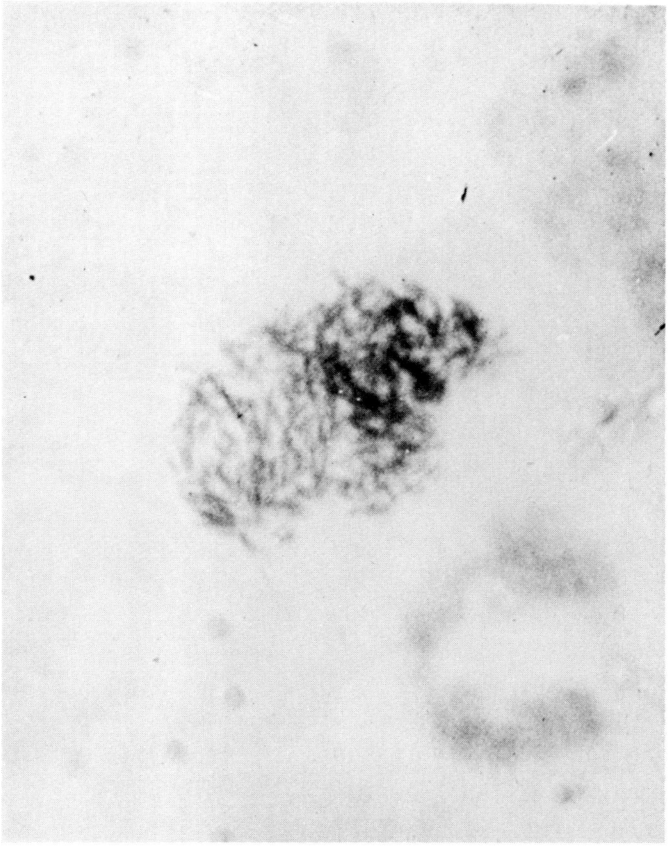

Fig. 25. Photomicrograph, leprosy bacilli in peripheral blood. Ziehl-Nielsen stain of defibrinated venous blood prior to therapy. Cluster may represent bacilli in remnant of a phagocytic leukocyte. Polymorphonuclear leukocyte nucleus is adjacent. Original magnification 1000X. (Pt.1)

PATIENT 2

A 26-Year-Old Male of Mestizo Extraction.

Spontaneous improvement was observed before treatment was started, and he continued to improve with sulfone therapy. Leukopenia and diffuse granulomatosis were present (Fig. 26). Tentative Diagnosis: Dimorphous leprosy. Final Diagnosis: Tuberculoid leprosy.

History. The patient had been in good health until thirteen months prior to his arrival at the Clinical Center. His first symptoms were "numbness" in the distal portions of his extremities. At the same time, he noticed hypochromic macules on his skin, which later turned red, then disappeared over a three-month period. He felt well thereafter until four months prior to admission to the Center, when he experienced sudden onset of fever and chills, arthralgias, myalgias, thirst, anorexia and loss of 4.5 kg of body weight. Reddened anesthetic macules appeared on his face and extremities, and, later, on his trunk (Figs. 27, 29). One month after that onset he again became aware of anesthesia in the distal portions of his extremities, when he burned himself with a cigarette. He developed weakness in the muscles of his hands (Fig. 28), lower legs and feet, and had difficulty closing his right eye (Fig. 30). He noticed alopecia in the macules, epistaxis, conjunctivitis, and decreasing vision in the right eye.

Two months prior to his arrival at the Center, the patient was examined at the Centro Dermatologico Pascua, where a diagnosis of leprosy was made. Acid-fast bacilli were found in cutaneous and nasal scrapings, and a lepromin skin test was "negative." Symptomatic treatment was begun with hydroxychloroquine, vitamins and iron tablets, and he received a short course of penicillin therapy. This patient had experienced poor vision in the right eye since childhood. He vaguely recalled prolonged illnesses in childhood and believed he may have had fevers at that time.

Epidemiological Data. The patient was born on a small farm in the eastern part of the state of Michoacan, Mexico, about 70 miles west of Mexico City. He lived in Guadalajara, Jalisco, as a child, and spent six months in the United States as a laborer, in

Los Angeles. He had lived with an aunt and uncle in Mexico City for the past seven years, working as an auto parts salesman. Another aunt was definitely known to have leprosy, and it was thought that a deceased grandmother had had leprosy. An invalid sister whom he had not seen for many years was reported to have had red cutaneous macules and fevers as a child. His father, mother, and seven brothers were all well.

Hospitalization at the Clinical Center (Fig. 31). The patient was observed for two months (Study Period I), during which time he was free of fever but complained of myalgias, insomnia and conjunctivitis in the right eye. Symptomatic therapy with aspirin, sedatives and methyl cellulose eye-drops gradually brought considerable relief from these symptoms. However, he remained unable to dress or feed himself because of weakness in the intrinsic musculature of the hands.

His erythrocyte sedimentation rate (ESR) was usually within the normal range, except following his renal biopsy. However, occasional spontaneous elevations in the ESR were observed, with a maximum value of 80, as outlined in Table 9. His white blood cell count was 2,900 at the time of his admission, and he demonstrated a persistent leukopenia during the entire hospitalization. Abnormalities in x-rays are illustrated in Figs. 32–34, and histopathologic features are shown in Figs. 35–40.

He was found to have a few acid-fast bacilli in association with giant cells and granulomas in the biopsy of a hyperchromic anesthetic macule (Table 4). A few acid-fast bacilli were also present in one of three bone marrow aspirations. No acid-fast bacilli were found in any other specimens of tissues or body secretions, except in one fecal specimen, a finding which was not thought to be significant.

Giant cells and granulomas were present in a lymph node and in the liver biopsy specimen, although bacilli were not observed in these biopsies. Atrophy, fibrosis and decreased spermatogenesis were seen in the biopsies of the testicles, and urinary ketosteroid excretion was less than normal in five out of seven 24-hour collections.

His neuromuscular abnormalities were severe, demonstrated by anesthesia of 23 percent of the body surface along with a decrease in muscular strength to 85 percent of normal. Healed chorioretinitis was present bilaterally, and was especially severe in the right eye, where visual acuity was diminished (20/200)

(Table 8). Studies of the etiology of chorioretinitis revealed a positive toxoplasmin dye titer (greater than 1:1000) and a positive tuberculin skin test.

Although many organs and systems were abnormal, the rarity of bacilli in the biopsy specimens made it impossible to determine which of his abnormalities were due to leprosy. A slight but definite clinical improvement was observed during the two months of observation in Study Period I.

Following the two month observation period, specific antileprosy chemotherapy was administered for five months. The period of therapy was called Study Period II. DDS was begun at a dose of 50 mg every two days, and increased to 100 mg per day over a six-week period, as shown in Fig. 31. A reticulocytosis developed while he was receiving DDS, to a maximum value of 4.1 percent (Fig. 31 and Table 9). He was found to have a shortening of the Cr^{51} red blood cell half-life to 18 days; the normal value in this laboratory was 28 days (Fig. 41). The increased hemolysis of red cells could not be definitely ascribed to any single cause, in the absence of pre-treatment Cr^{51} studies. However, the appearance of reticulocytosis while on DDS therapy suggested that hemolysis was at least partly a manifestation of sulfone toxicity.

The serum proteins showed a decrease in both albumin and globulin concentration during the period of DDS therapy (Fig. 31 and Table 7) but all values were within the normal range; the significance of this slight change is not clear. At the end of the treatment period he had developed some reossification in the bones of his hands, with diminution in the size of lytic areas which had been observed there (Figs. 33 and 34).

Specimens of skin and nasal mucosa failed to reveal bacilli during the entire period of DDS therapy, although one bone marrow specimen contained a few organisms, as described above. His lepromin skin test became "positive" and — inexplicably — his tuberculin skin test became "negative" after five months of DDS therapy. His skin lesions became less prominent as a more normal color returned to the skin (Fig. 42).

The ova of *Hymenolepis nana* and *Trichuris trichiura* were intermittently recovered from his feces during his hospitalization, but these parasites had disappeared at the conclusion of Study Period II.

During therapy, sensation returned to many of the previously anesthetic macules; only 20 percent of the body surface was anesthetic. Muscular power also improved; the final examination revealed strength estimated at 91 percent of normal. With return of muscular function, and with physical therapy, he improved in his ability to care for himself, although he continued to have severe weakness in the intrinsic muscles of the right hand.

Physical and occupational therapy gave this young man tremendous support. His disease appeared to be evolving into a quiescent granulomatous process without bacteria present — similar to "the burnt out case" of Graham Greene (1961). Whether or not he would be able to maintain himself in economic independence after his return to Mexico was doubtful, however, for his dominant hand had apparently suffered irreparable neurologic damage.

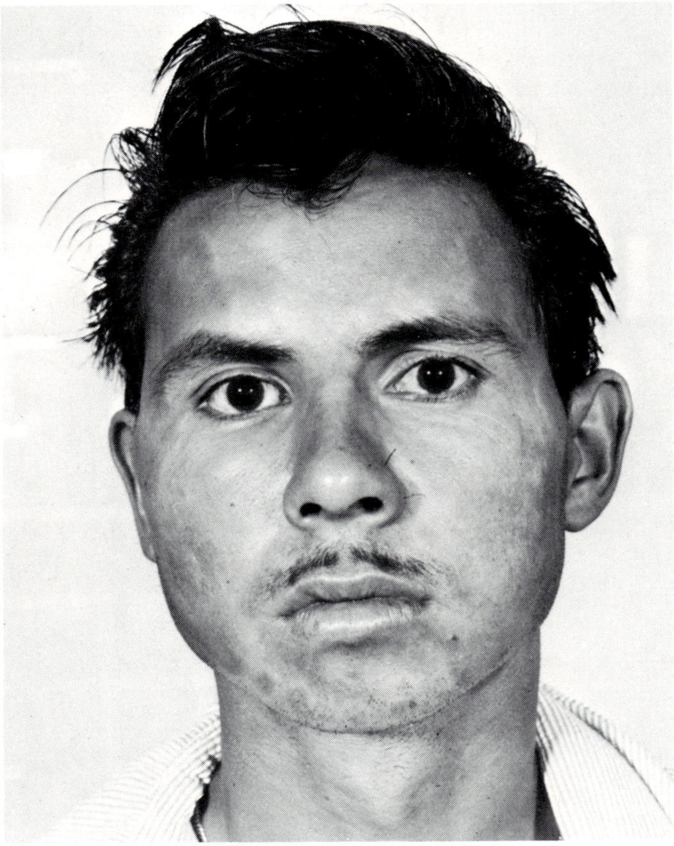

Fig. 26. A 26-year-old man initially believed to have dimorphous leprosy; rapid decrease in bacterial counts led to diagnosis of tuberculoid leprosy. Face shows hyperchromic macules with dysesthesia. (Pt. 2)

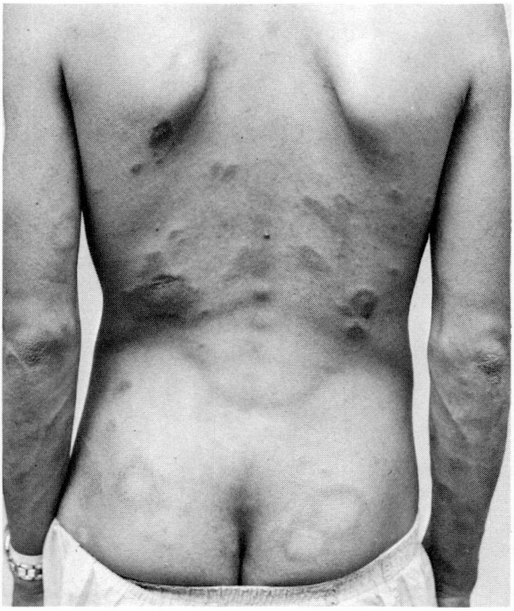

Fig. 27. Macules on back, buttocks and arms. Older lesions have hypochromic central areas, are hypesthetic, not tender; newer lesions painful and tender, pinprick perception diminished. (Pt. 2)

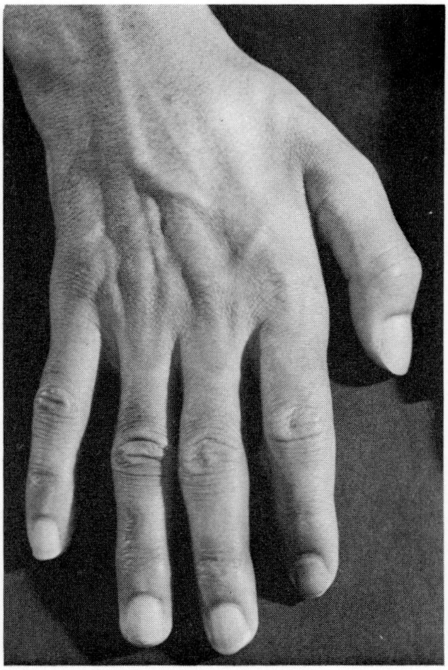

Fig. 28. Atrophy of intrinsic musculature hands due to ulnar and median nerves. Atrophy of the thumb "web space" prominent bilaterally due to loss of nerve to first dorsal interosseous muscle. (Pt. 2)

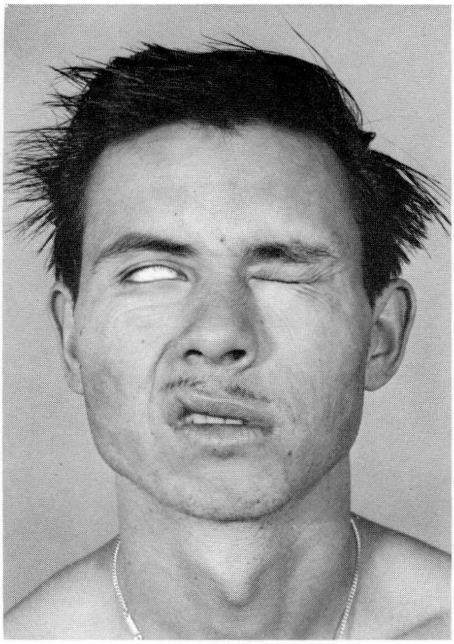

Fig. 30. Lagophthalmos, caused by facial nerve palsy; inability to close eye. Patient attempts to compensate by elevating angle of lip. Right eye dry, painful, with chronic conjunctivitis. (Pt. 2)

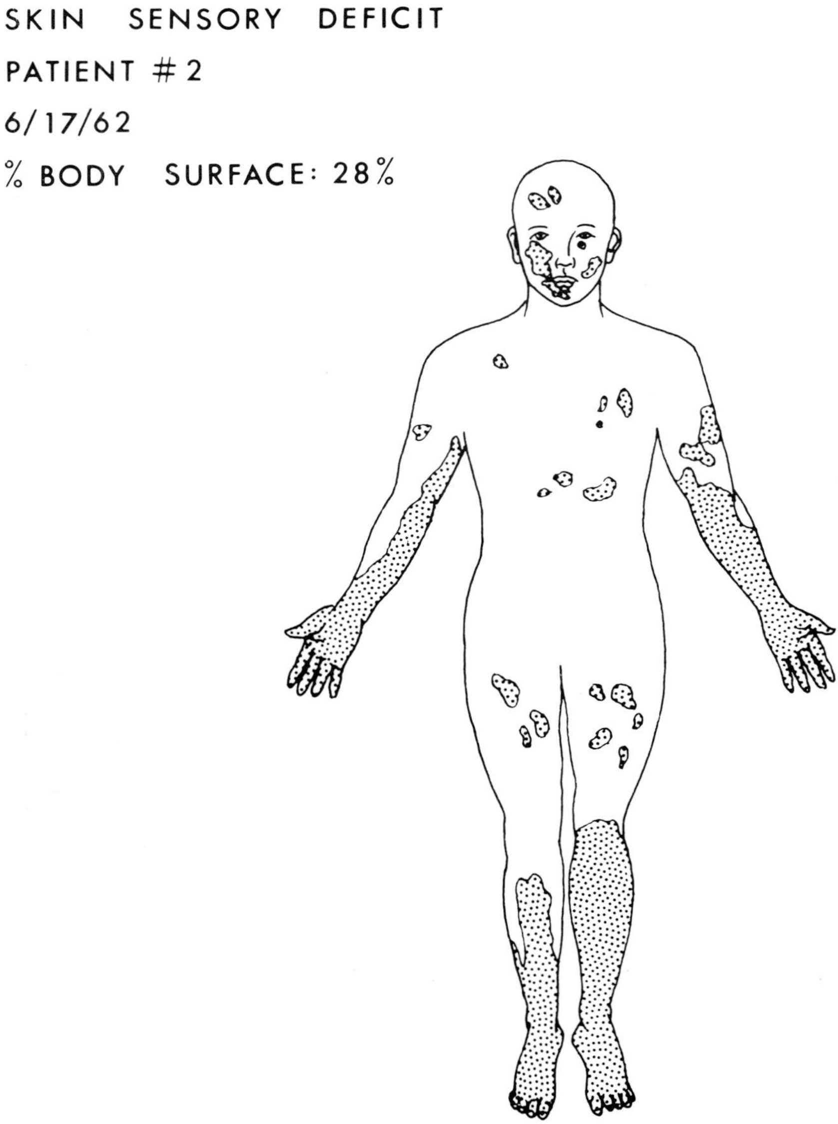

Fig. 29. Skin sensory deficit. 28% of body surface. (Pt. 2)

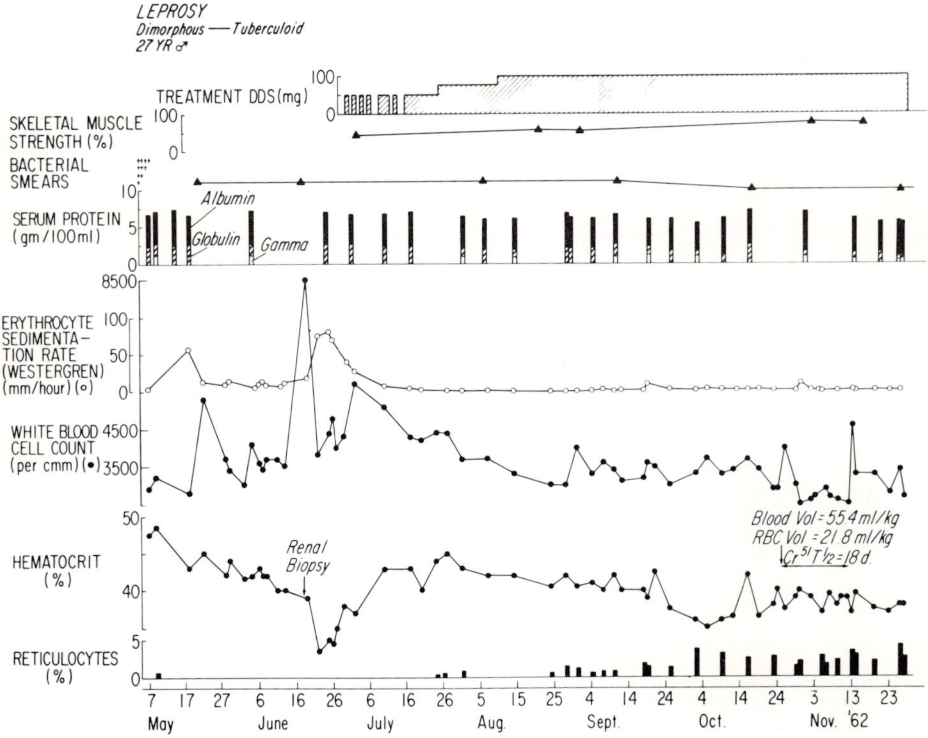

Fig. 31. Clinical Course Chart. Gradual improvement during hospitalization: rise in skeletal muscular strength, decline in bacteria in skin scrapings and serum globulin. Low hematocrit, diminished red cell survival, and elevated reticulocyte count while receiving DDS suggest a mild degree of hemolytic anemia. (Pt. 2)

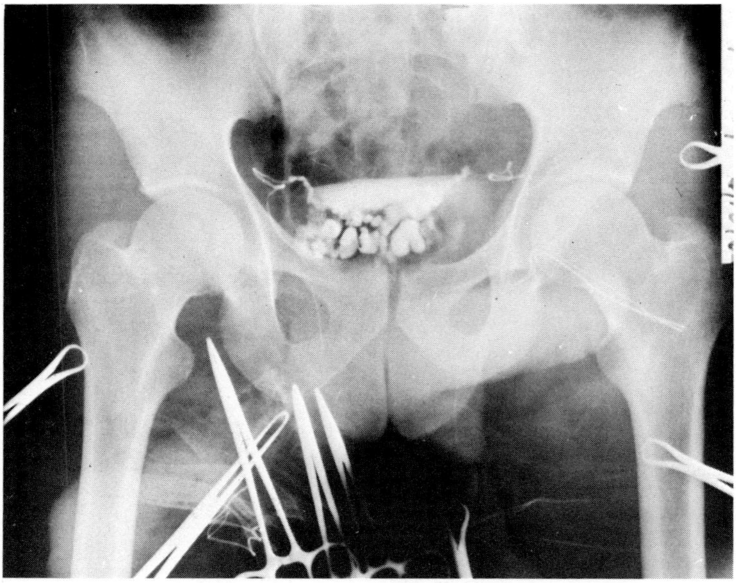

Fig. 32. X-ray, seminal vesiculogram. Dilatation and delayed emptying of seminal vesicles is demonstrated, five minutes after Hypaque® injection. (Pt. 2)

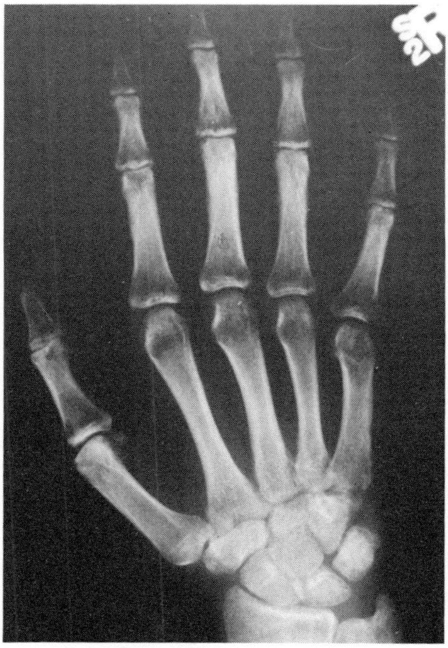

Fig. 33. X-ray, hands. Diffuse demineralization of bones at time of admission: no evidence of osteitis or osteomyelitis. (Pt. 2)

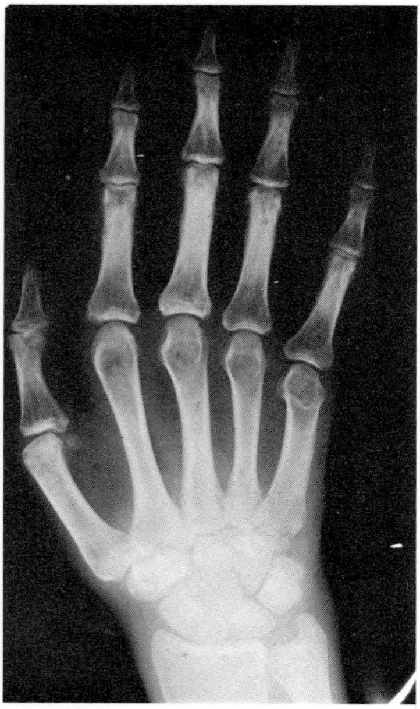

Fig. 34. X-ray, hands. Film taken six months after Fig. 33. Remineralization has occurred following sulfone therapy. (Pt. 2)

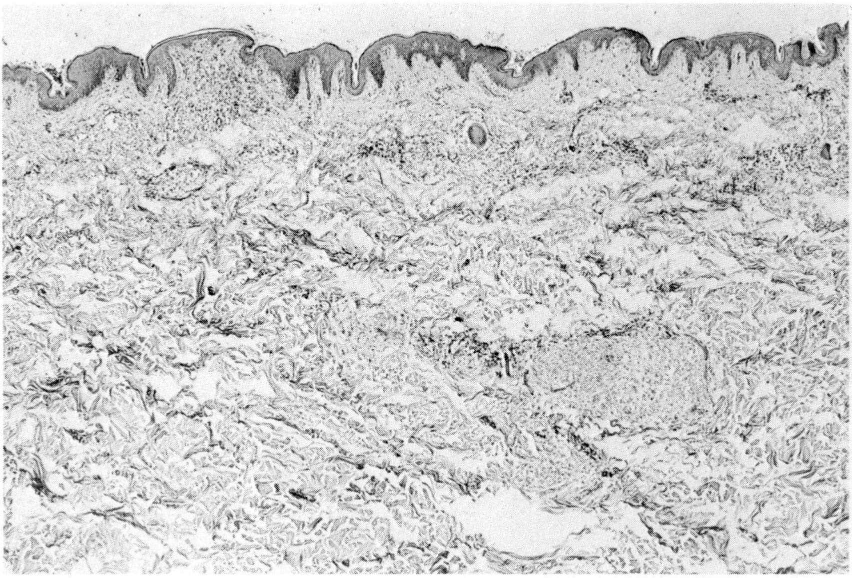

Fig. 35. Photomicrograph, skin. Active tuberculoid macule; indurated, painful, erythematous, anesthetic to pin prick. Dermal inflammation apparent in lymphocytes, macrophages, and Langhans giant cells. Under oil immersion, Fite stain of same specimen showed acid-fast bacilli in subcutaneous nerves. (Pt. 2)

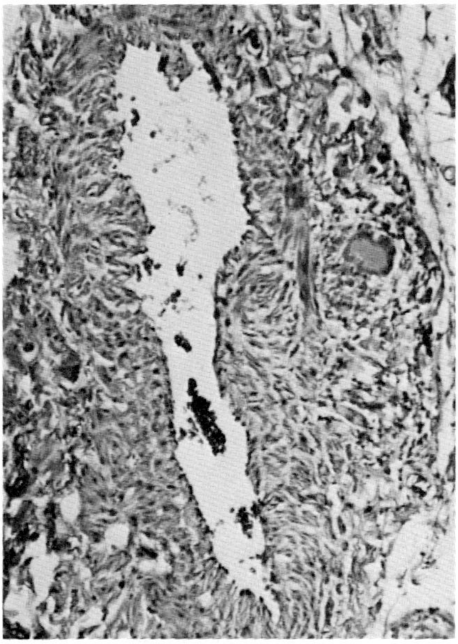

Fig. 36. Photomicrograph, skin. Another area of tuberculoid macule seen in Fig. 35 revealed granulomatus arteritis with proliferation of intima, medial necrosis, and giant cells. No acid-fast bacilli found with Fite stain. H & E stain, 105X. (Pt. 2)

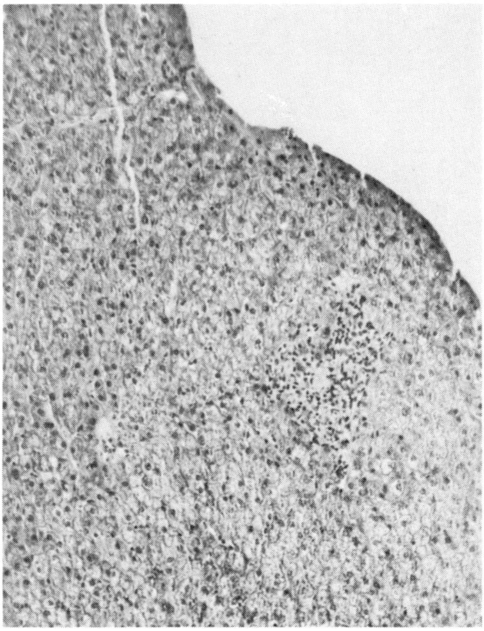

Fig. 37. Photomicrograph, liver. Biopsy obtained prior to therapy. Small granulomas with macrophages and giant cells. No acid-fast bacilli. H & E stain, 105X. (Pt. 2)

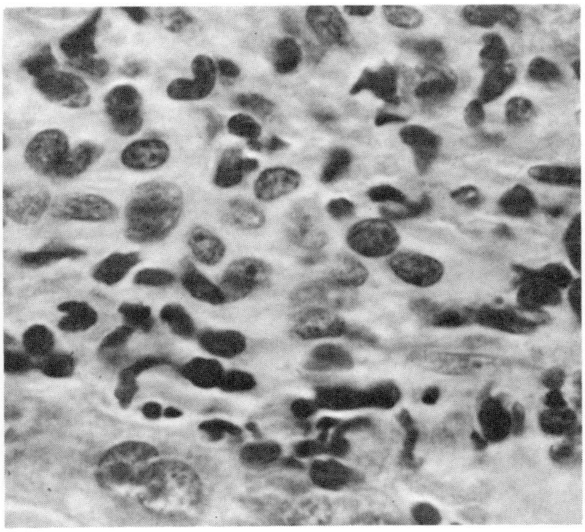

Fig. 38. Photomicrograph, liver. Higher magnification of one of granulomas seen in Fig. 37. H & E stain, 778X (Pt. 2)

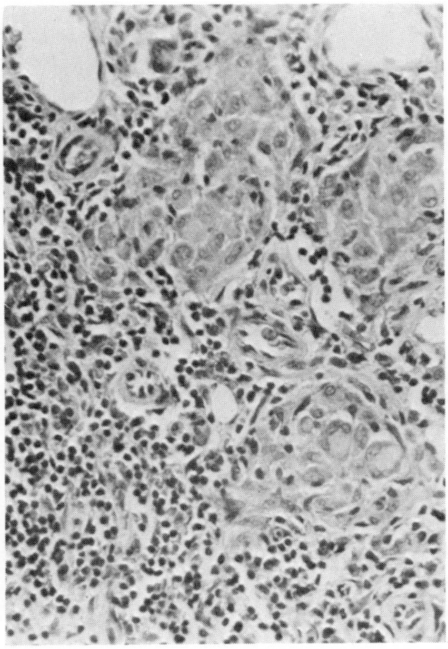

Fig. 39. Photomicrograph, inguinal lymph node. A large firm node biopsied prior to therapy. No acid-fast bacilli present, but shows multiple granulomas with giant cells, large macrophages. H & E stain, 225X (Pt. 2)

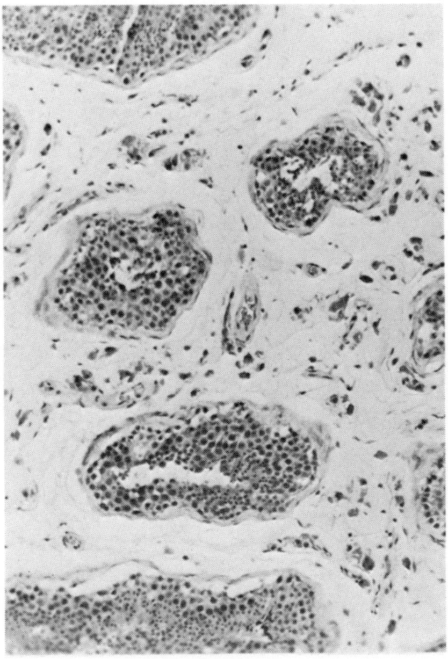

Fig. 40. Photomicrograph, testicle. Enlarged, firm, slightly tender; biopsied prior to therapy. Diminished spermatogenesis, interstitial edema, and fibrosis apparent. No acid-fast bacilli seen with Fite stain. H & E stain, 95X. (Pt. 2)

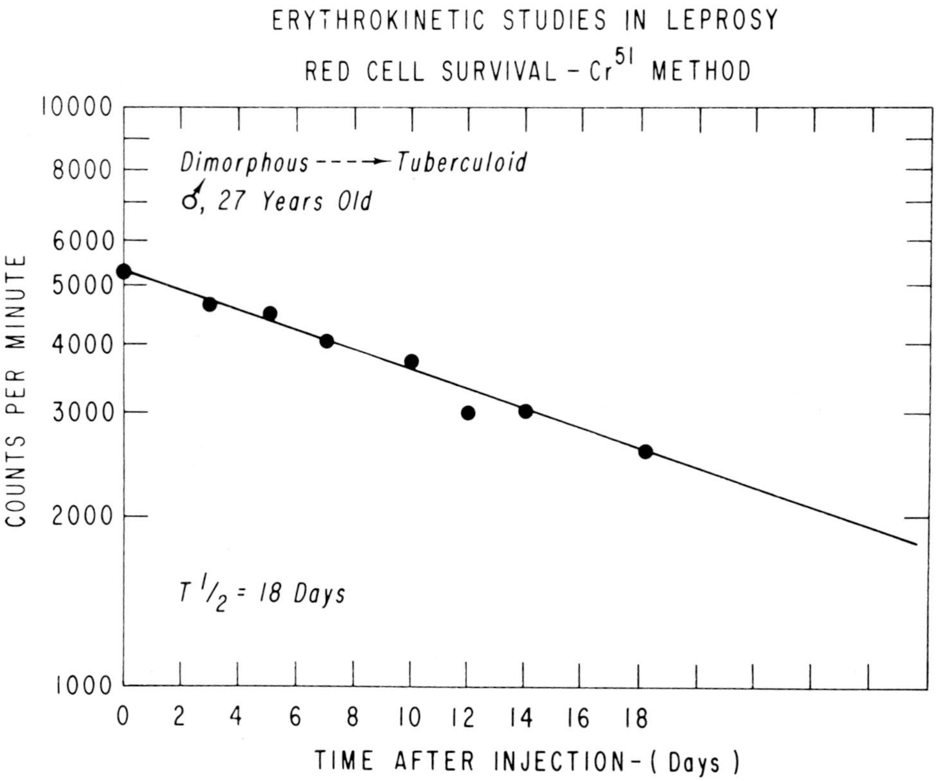

Fig. 41. Hemolytic anemia studied with Cr^{51} RBC labelling. Patient developed reticulocytosis after three months DDS therapy. Hematocrit 37. Reticulocyte count 2.2%. (Pt. 2)

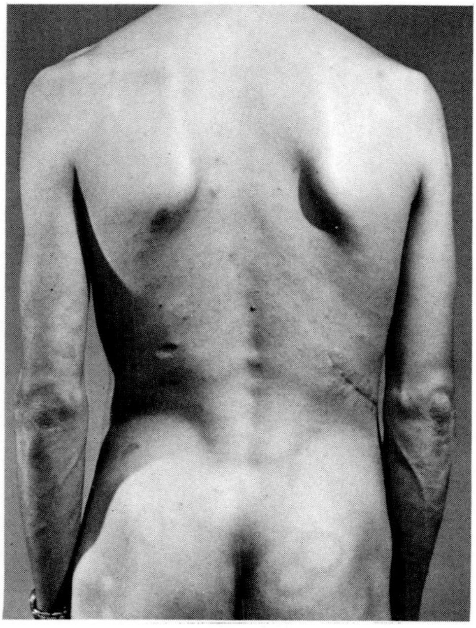

Fig. 42. Back and buttocks six months after initial photograph (Fig. 27). After four months of sulfone therapy reactive macules had somewhat subsided. Classification "tuberculoid" at this time. (Pt. 2)

PATIENT 3

A 14-Year-Old Male of Mestizo Extraction

Virtually asymptomatic when first seen. During treatment he developed extensive functional abnormalities, even though he was bacteriologically improved (Figs. 43, 44). Tentative Diagnosis: Indeterminate leprosy. Final Diagnosis: Lepromatous leprosy, with lepra reaction, associated with bacteriologic improvement.

History. The patient had never been ill, and only came to the attention of physicians as the result of an epidemiologic survey of his family. The survey was performed because his mother was found to have lepromatous leprosy. In retrospect he recalled that he had had "numbness" of his fingers for about two and one-half years, gradually progressing to involve his entire arms. He had also noticed several small hypochromic macules on his body which developed partial alopecia. He had never had fever, muscular pain or any other symptoms of generalized disease. He had worked regularly as a tailor's apprentice until he was brought to the United States for study.

When he was examined at the Instituto Dermatologico, Guadalajara, he was found to have slight muscular weakness in the forearms and hands, and his earlobes were enlarged and erythematous. Additional hypochromic macules were discovered on the buttocks and chin. Nasal and cutaneous scrapings failed to reveal leprosy bacilli, but a skin biopsy showed a few organisms in enlarged dermal nerves. He exhibited a "negative" response to intradermal lepromin.

Epidemiological Data. The patient's birthplace and residence is in Guadalajara, where he lives with his father, mother and five siblings. Guadalajara is Mexico's second largest city (population 700,000 in 1962) and is located 290 miles northwest of Mexico City at an altitude of 5,200 feet. The climate is warm and pleasant, and the city is a major tourist center.

The patient's mother (Fig. 45) was referred to the Instituto Dermatologico for a minor dermatologic problem two years previously. At that time she was recognized as having lepromatous leprosy. Since her diagnosis was established she has taken DDS and DPT in low doses. She has never had any fever or acute reactions. The patient's father and siblings, all of whom live at home with him, are apparently in good health.

Hospitalization at the Clinical Center (Fig. 46). The patient was observed during Study Period I, which lasted for two months. During this time his clinical condition appeared to be stable. It was discovered that leprosy bacilli were present in greater numbers in his skin biopsies than had been the case only three months previously in Mexico (Figs. 47 and 48). Areas of skin which were grossly normal revealed many organisms in the dermis, especially in nerves and near dermal appendages, where globi were seen.

Biopsy of the liver (Fig. 49) revealed a small number of acid-fast bacilli in portal areas; a lymph node (Fig. 50) was seen to contain many free acid-fast bacilli and globi (Table 4). Nasal and cutaneous scrapings continued to reveal only a few organisms, however.

He had no anemia, leukocytosis or elevation of the erythrocyte sedimentation rate. His total serum globulin and gamma globulin levels were slightly elevated (3.9 and 1.5 gm per 100 ml respectively).

The patient showed evidence of a mild peripheral neuropathy on electromyogram. He demonstrated anesthesia or hypesthesia on 26 percent of his body surface (Fig. 51); his skeletal muscle strength was diminished to 93.5 percent of normal. Analysis of his semen showed moderate abnormalities (Table 14), and his serum carotene and Vitamin A levels were in the low-normal range (70 and 48 gamma per 100 ml respectively).

The elevation of alkaline phosphatase to 30 units was thought to be due to adolescent osteogenesis. His adrenal, renal and serologic tests were all normal, and the bone marrow contained no leprosy bacilli. Because of the leprosy bacilli in skin, lymph nodes, and liver, his condition was believed to be more serious than was originally apparent. He was reclassified as "early lepromatous."

In Study Period II, lasting three months, the patient received anti-leprosy chemotherapy (DDS) for the first time. He received 50 mg per day for two weeks, 75 mg per day for one week, and 100 mg per day for the next three months. He remained free of fever, and his only symptoms were persistent anesthesia of the extremities. Only 10 percent of his body surface demonstrated abnormalities of sensation at the close of this study period, and his skeletal muscle strength increased to 99 percent of normal. He showed a slight decrease in his serum globulin and gamma globulin levels (mean values 2.9 and 0.9 gm per 100 ml, respectively).

A granulomatous reaction to intradermal lepromin was observed; a 3 mm nodule was present three weeks after lepromin was injected. Giant cells containing leprosy bacilli were seen on histologic examination of this nodule (Fig. 52). The nodule was still less than 5 mm in size, however, and was therefore described as "negative" clinically.

During therapy (Study Period II) the patient developed a moderate degree of anemia, the hematocrit falling to 33.5 (Table 9). The anemia was believed not to be due to the withdrawal of blood specimens for laboratory tests: less blood was removed than during Study Period I, when his hematocrit remained stable. Reticulocytosis was observed (maximum 3.4 percent), and the anemia was tentatively ascribed to a hemolytic reaction to DDS.

Another disturbing phenomenon present during the latter part of Study Period II was the absence of a rise in plasma corticoids during infusion of ACTH, although a normal rise in urinary corticoid excretion was observed (18.6 mg in 24 hours). Increased numbers of acid-fast bacilli were recovered in scrapings of skin and nasal mucosa and in the liver biopsy specimen (Fig. 53).

After three months of DDS therapy the patient gradually developed a progressive dermatitis (Fig. 54), followed by fever and peripheral neuritis. Sensory abnormalities developed on 50 percent of the body surface and muscular strength decreased to 72 percent of normal. With the onset of the fever and dermatitis, which will subsequently be referred to as "the reaction," DDS therapy was discontinued.

The remainder of this patient's hospitalization, which lasted for four months, has been called Study Period III. The treatment during this period consisted of short courses of prednisone and the antileprosy drug DPT (Fig. 46). With prednisone dosage of 20 mg per day, fever and malaise diminished; relief was often obtained from smaller doses of prednisone. The dermatitis appeared to improve gradually during steroid therapy, but muscular weakness became progressively more severe (Fig. 55).

Near the end of Period III the patient developed a mild left lagophthalmos (Fig. 56). He developed enlargement of the earlobes, lips and nasal alae — "leonine facies" — prior to the institution of prednisone therapy; these features are shown in Fig. 57. Although his appearance suggested an increased proliferation of organisms, cutaneous scrapings and biopsies of skin and earlobe (Figs. 58 and 59) did not reveal increased numbers of bacilli. The density of organisms in the skin scrapings gradually diminished during the remainder of the hospitalization. No bacilli were recovered from skin scrapings during the last two months of Study Period III, and only small numbers of bacilli were seen in lymph node biopsies and a bone marrow aspiration at that time.

Although the patient's bacterial status improved, he began to exhibit abnormalities in renal function. The abnormalities included elevation in BUN; decrease in PSP excretion, renal concentrating power and creatinine clearance; and the appearance of proteinuria and cylindruria. The dosage of DPT was reduced in view of the possibility that it could be causing renal toxicity.

The patient also developed hypochromic, microcytic anemia, a low reticulocyte count and a low serum iron. He had a normal iron binding capacity, but showed no improvement after two months' therapy with iron sulfate by mouth. The patient's anemia was investigated using Cr^{51} red cell labeling; normal half-life was shown to be present (Fig. 60). The blood volume was normal, but the red cell volume was diminished (Table 9). Hemolysis was thus ruled out as a significant cause of his anemia. These studies were performed after DDS had been discontinued and sulfone was not detectable in the patient's plasma. DDS did not appear, therefore, to have been the cause of the anemia in this patient, and no single cause was found.

Adrenal function was studied with two ACTH tests during Study Period III (Tables 12, 13). The first test was interpreted as showing decreased adrenal responsiveness. Two weeks later, the patient showed a rise in plasma and urinary 17OH corticosteroids to slightly above the normal range after an ACTH infusion. He thus appeared to demonstrate some adrenal response to ACTH, although not to the extent observed in Study Periods I and II. During Study Period III the total serum globulin levels once again became elevated.

This young man was an especially distressing problem in management, for in spite of good bacteriologic improvement and careful attempts to control his inflammatory reactions, he suffered severe abnormalities in many systems, some of which may have become irreversible.

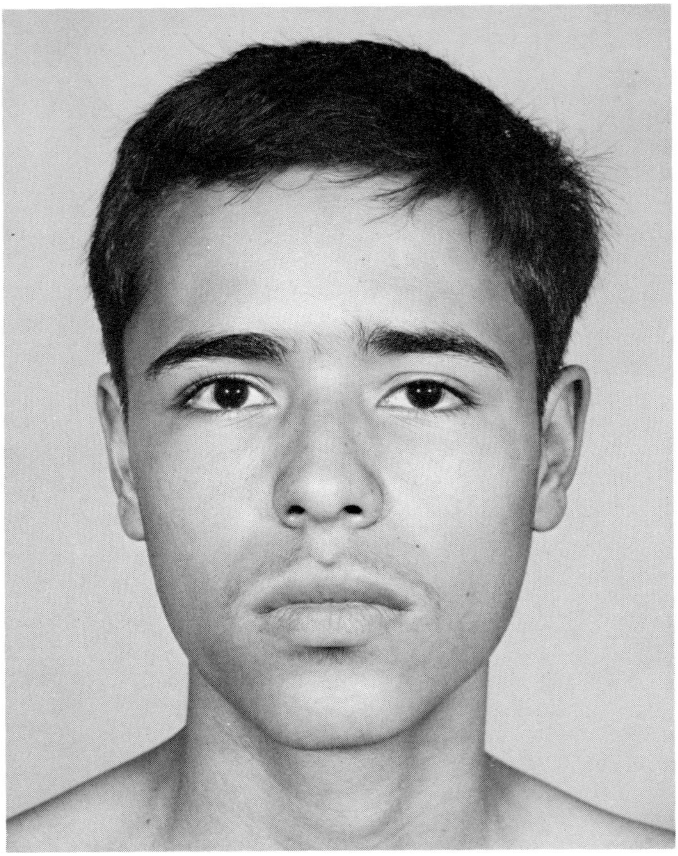

Fig. 43. A 14-year-old boy; only surface abnormalities were areas of slight hypochromic alteration on buttocks. Diminished sensation in buttock macules and on distal aspects of arms and legs. (Pt. 3)

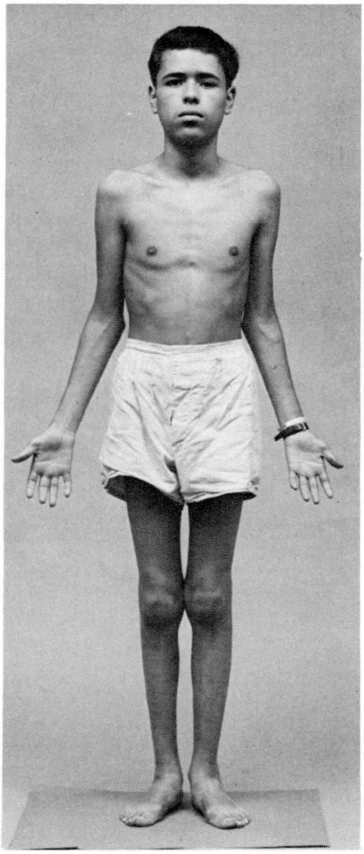

Fig. 44. Photograph taken four and one-half months after Fig. 43, following two and one-half months of sulfone therapy. Patient felt well, had gained weight, no new lesions apparent. Biopsy site on left forearm; antecubital veins enlarged due to venipunctures. (Pt. 3)

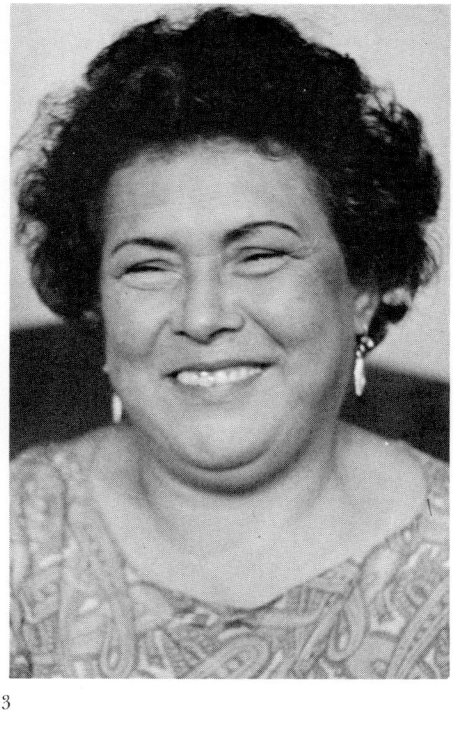

Fig. 45. Mother of patient 3, has lepromatous leprosy, is being treated with DDS. Like son, has extensive involvement by leprosy in absence of prominent symptoms and signs of disease.

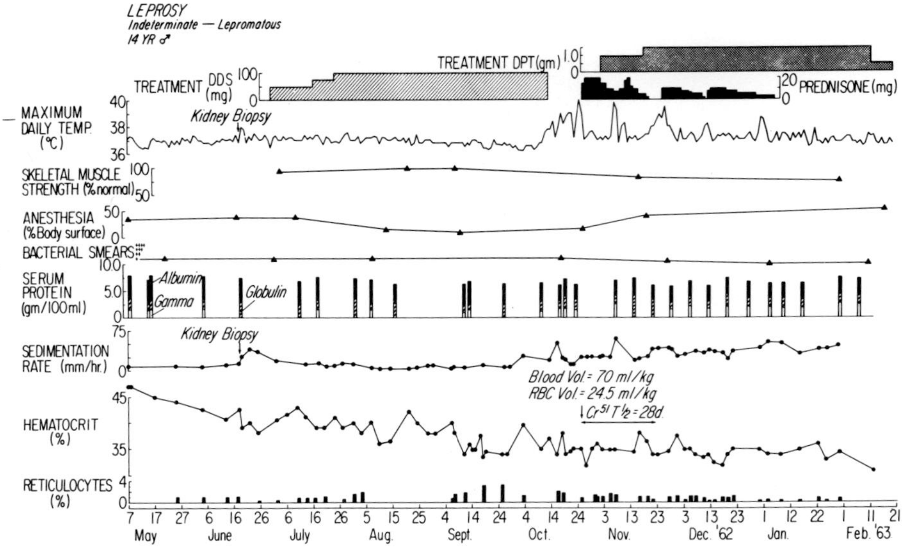

Fig. 46. Clinical Course Chart. Stable until therapy, then improvement followed by deterioration: fever, diminished strength and sensation. Elevation in gamma globulin and ESR, but bacterial smears improved as appearance worsened. Gradually became anemic without elevation in reticulocyte count. (Pt. 3)

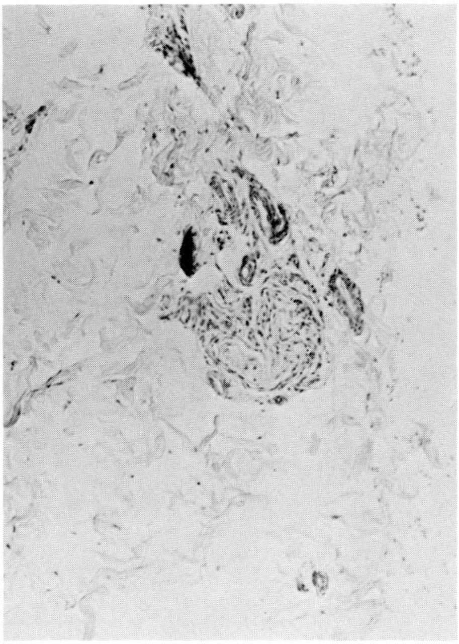

Fig. 47. Photomicrograph, skin, anesthetic macule. Slight enlargement of subcutaneous nerves, one of which is depicted here. Bacilli were in groups of two or three, not particularly numerous. H & E stain, 30X. (Pt. 3)

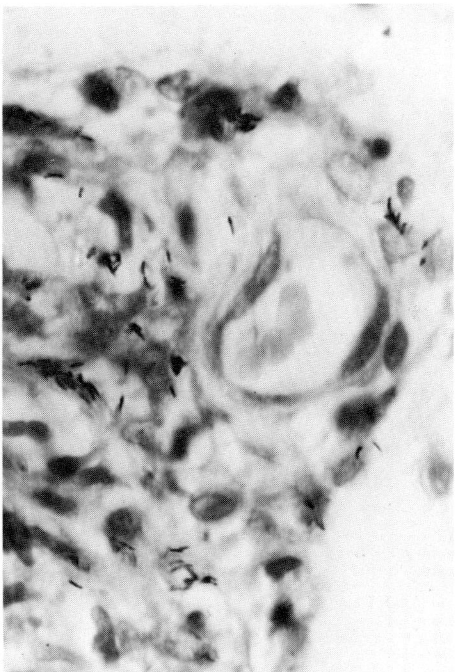

Fig. 48. Photomicrograph, skin, grossly normal. Large numbers of leprosy bacilli in subcutaneous tissues of "normal" skin two months after biopsy in Fig. 47. Normal texture and sensation but apparently disease now widely disseminated. Fite stain, 1010X. (Pt. 3)

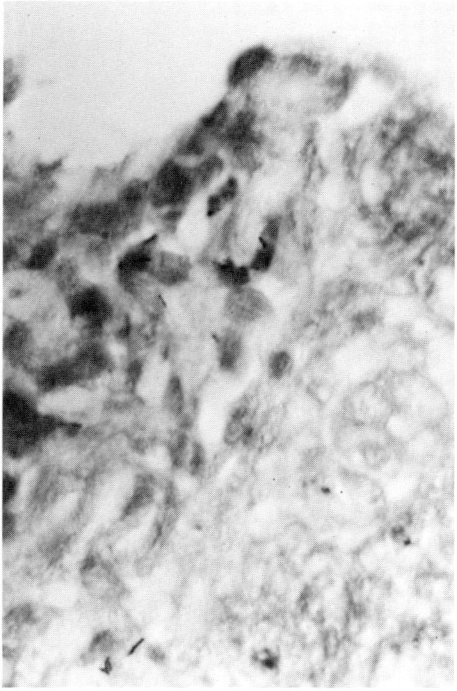

Fig. 49. Photomicrograph, liver. Acid-fast bacilli present in small numbers in portal areas; liver function tests normal, patient felt well. These organisms were first indication disease had become disseminated. Fite stain, 1010X. (Pt. 3)

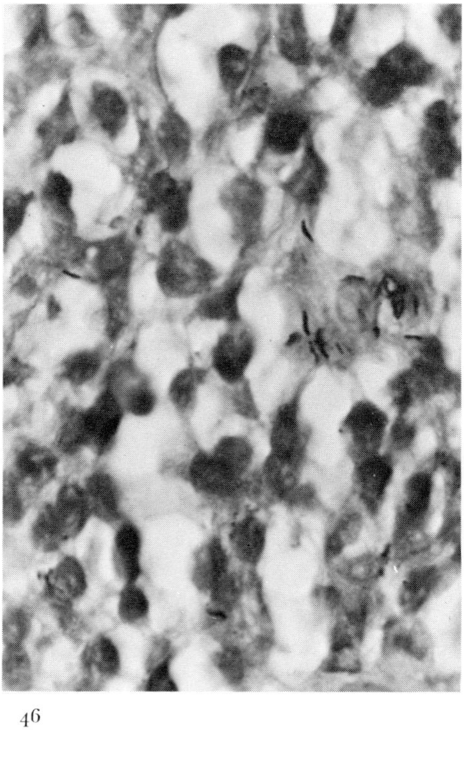

Fig. 50. Photomicrograph, inguinal lymph node. Architecture of node essentially normal, but globi seen; acid-fast organisms present in many fields. Further evidence that disease now "lepromatous" instead of "indeterminate." Fite stain, 1010X. (Pt. 3)

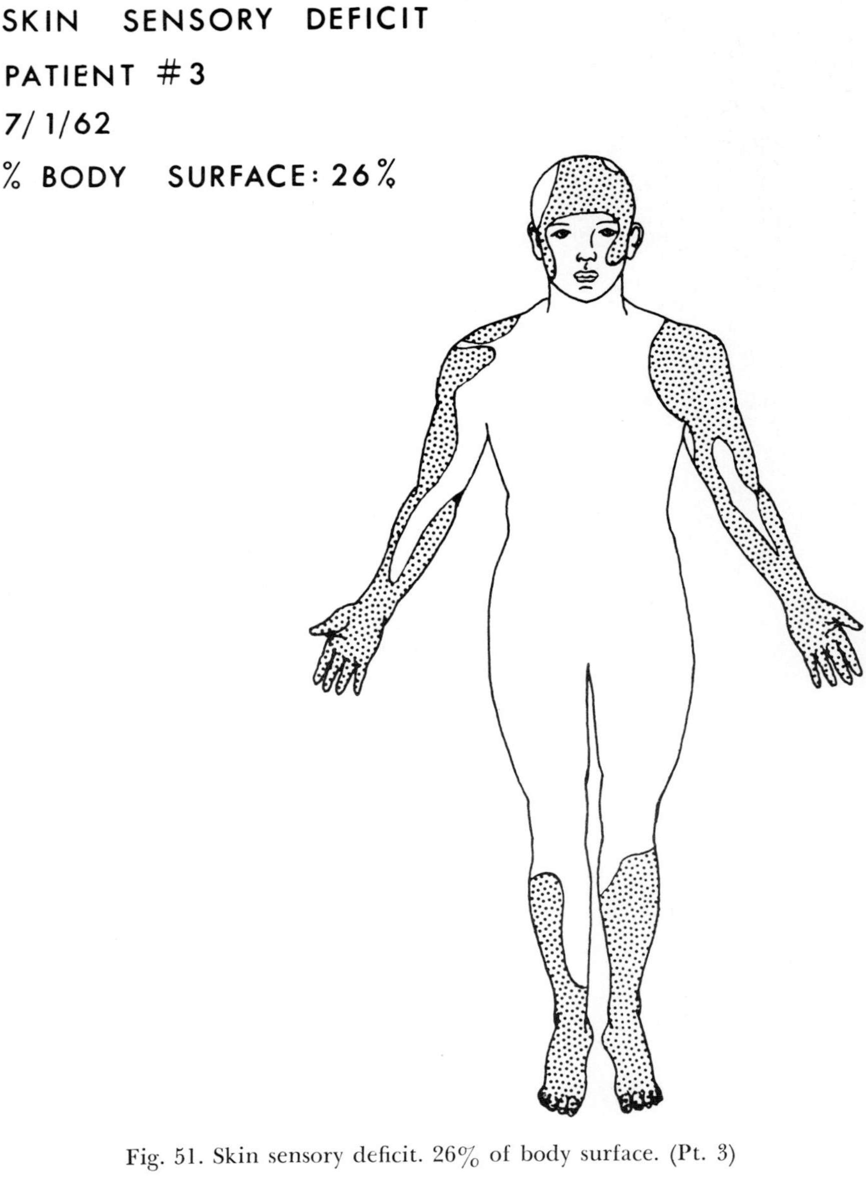

Fig. 51. Skin sensory deficit. 26% of body surface. (Pt. 3)

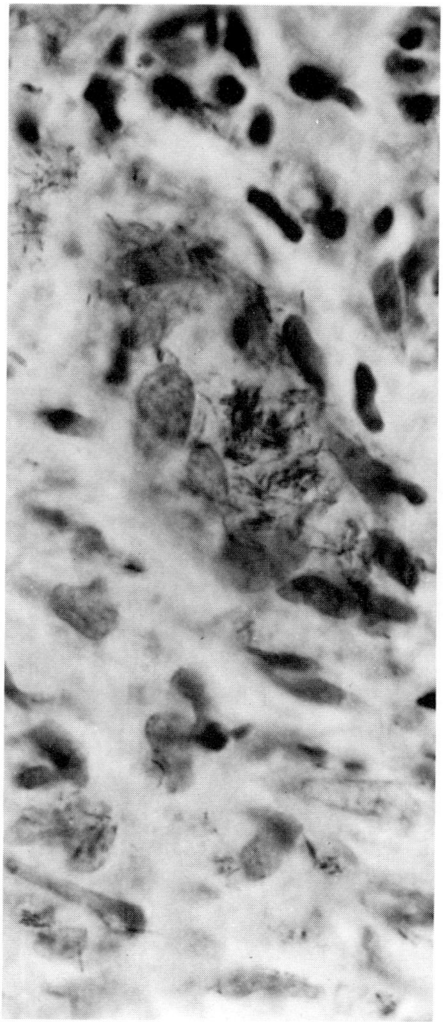

Fig. 52. Photomicrograph, lepromin skin test. Incorporation of injected bacilli into macrophages and giant cells. Histology is similar to that of "positive" lepromin reactions, presumably reflects immune cellular response by patient. Fite stain, 1252X. (Pt. 3)

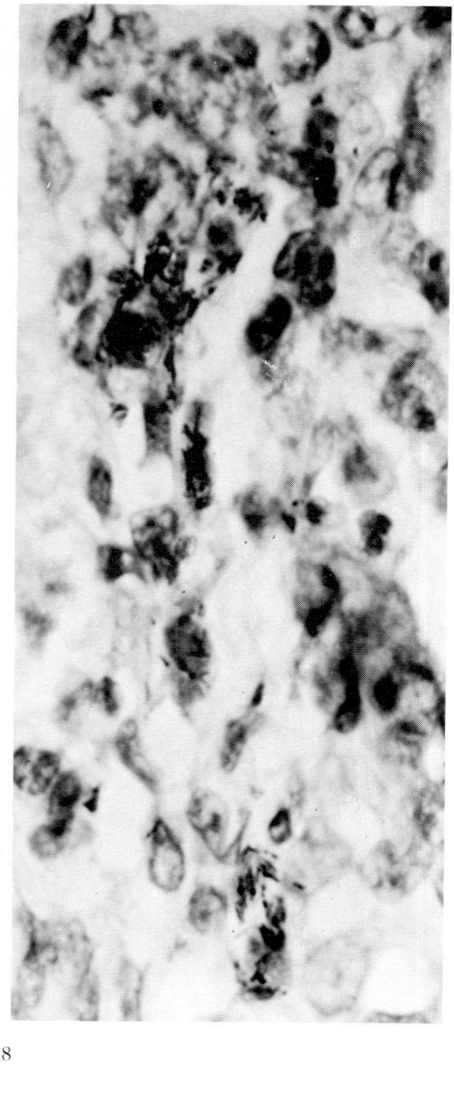

Fig. 53. Photomicrograph, liver, second biopsy. Portal areas contain increased lymphocytes and macrophages, globi, and clusters of bacilli. Increased number of organisms in liver may represent phagocytosis of dead and dying organisms or proliferation of organisms in deep tissues of body. Fite stain, 1273X. (Pt. 3)

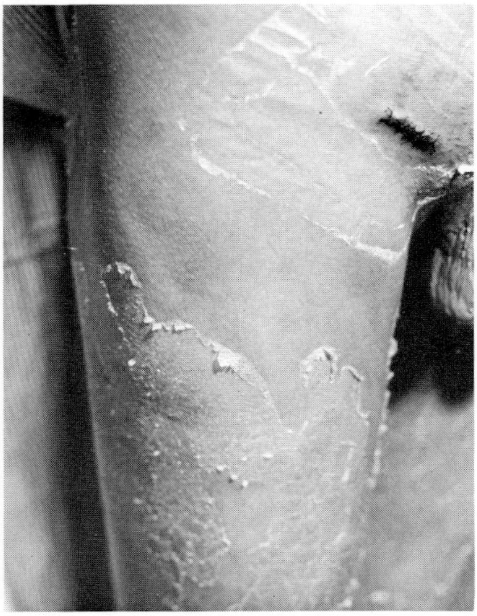

Fig. 54. Exfoliative dermatitis of right thigh, six months after admission. Sulfone therapy discontinued one month before photograph because of fever and dermatitis. Inguinal node biopsy at this time showed only a few acid-fast bacilli. (Pt. 3)

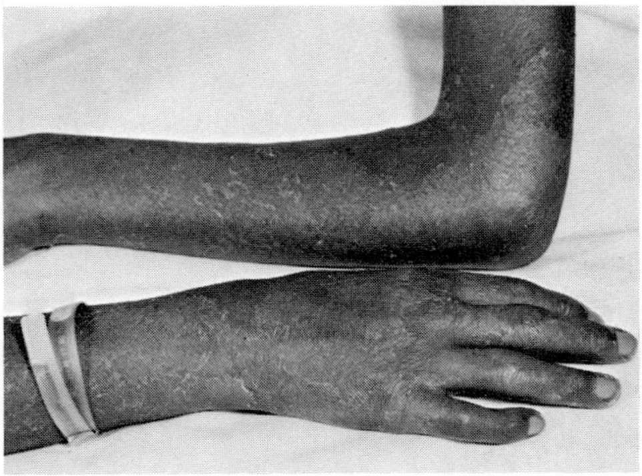

Fig. 55. Hand, during febrile reaction, two weeks after photograph, Fig. 54. Pain and neuropathy present, all muscle groups affected, atrophy of thenar eminences. X-rays showed demineralization. (Pt. 3)

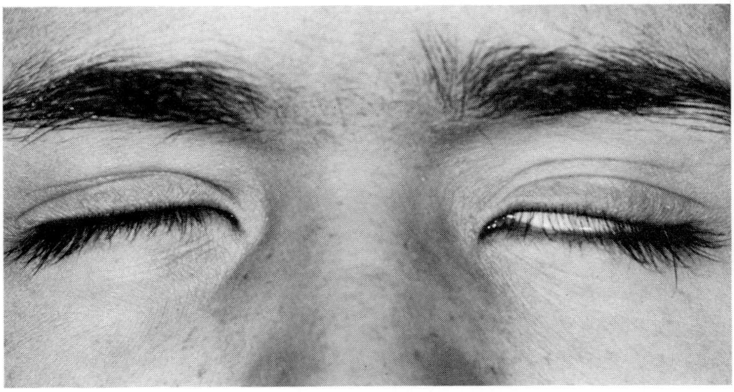

Fig. 56. Lagophthalmos of left eye, during febrile reaction. Sulfones discontinued three and one-half months before photograph. Had received prednisone therapy; muscular weakness unimproved although temperature normal. (Pt. 3)

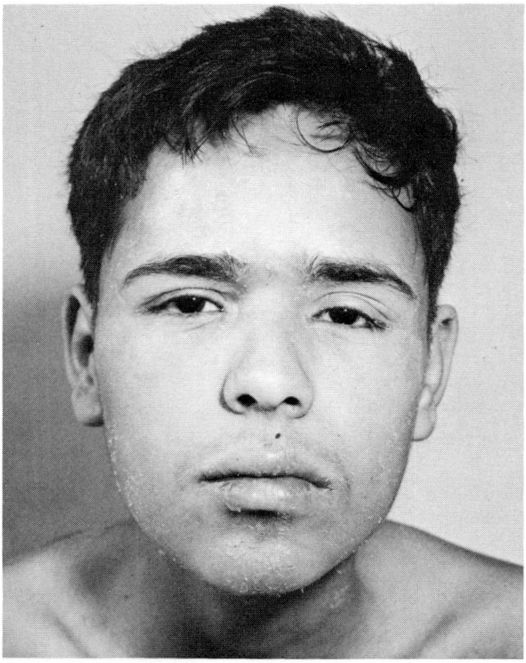

Fig. 57. Facial edema, prominent in ears, lips, nose, and eyelids, during febrile reaction. Photographed two months after cessation of sulfone therapy. Earlobe biopsy at this time showed few acid-fast bacilli. Chronic inflammation of dermis and subcutaneous tissues. (Pt. 3)

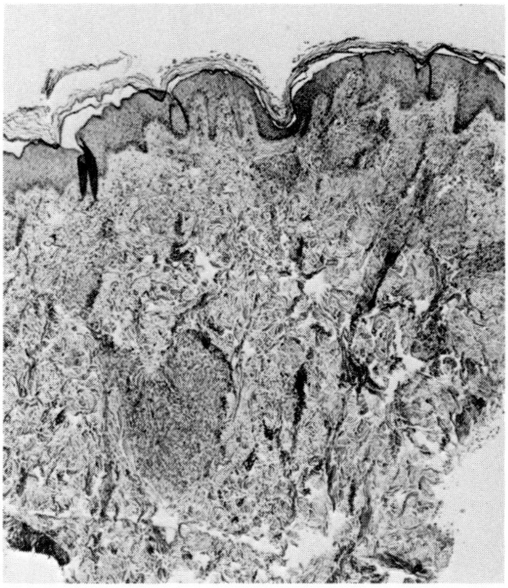

Fig. 58. Photomicrograph, skin, exfoliative dermatitis. Biopsy obtained during febrile reaction, Study Period III. Masses of chronic inflammatory cells have appearance of granulomata at this magnification. Fite stain, 27X. (Pt. 3)

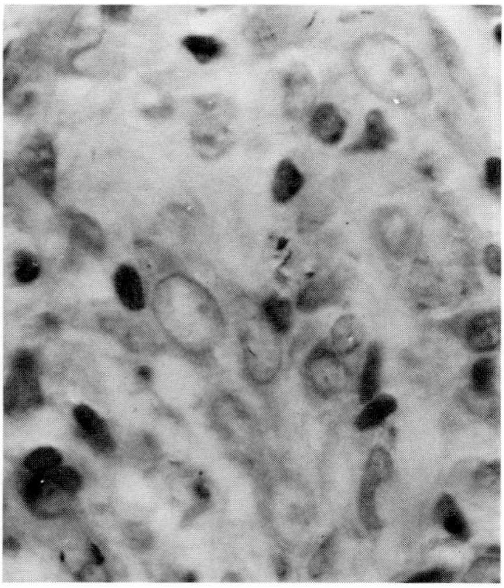

Fig. 59. Photomicrograph, skin, exfoliative dermatitis. Higher magnification of Fig. 58 shows a few leprosy bacilli, many macrophages, lymphocytes, plasma cells; no giant cells. Many areas contained no bacilli. Fite stain, 909X. (Pt. 3)

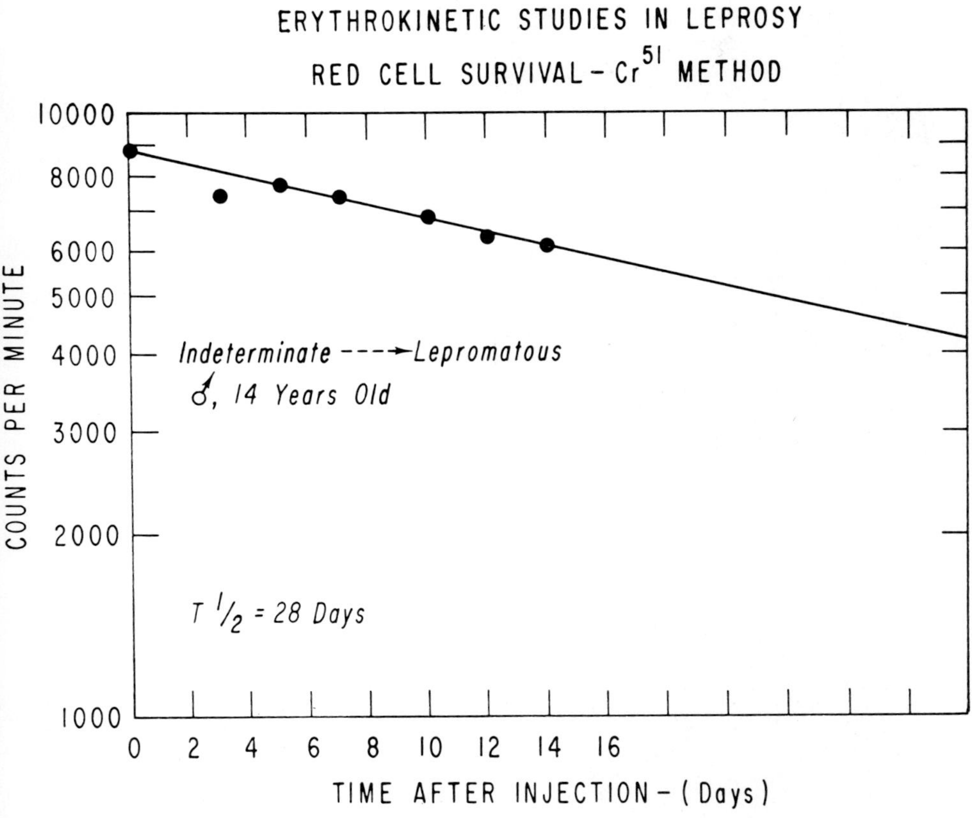

Fig. 60. Red cell survival curve obtained when patient was anemic, during febrile reaction of Study Period III. Normal Cr^{51} RBC T½ (28 days) ruled out hemolysis as cause of fall in hematocrit to 35. (Pt. 3)

PATIENT 4

A 22-Year-Old Male of Mestizo Extraction

Erythema nodosum, fever, weight loss and anemia recurred with cyclical periodicity (Figs. 61–65). Tentative Diagnosis: Lepromatous leprosy, with erythema nodosum phenomenon. Final Diagnosis: Same.

History. The patient was in excellent health until seven years prior to admission, when he first noticed hypochromic and hyperchromic macules on his legs and back. About four years prior to admission he began to have transient erythematous, tender nodules on his forearms, thighs, and left eyebrow, associated with fever and malaise. He was in good health between the febrile episodes, which confined him to bed, but was unable to meet his six-month military training obligation because of recurrent fever. He subsequently worked as a farmer and truck driver's assistant.

Because of recurrence of the nodules at approximately monthly intervals, and the development of persistent induration of the skin of his thighs, the patient consulted a doctor in his community. The doctor recognized the lesions as erythema nodosum, and referred the patient to the Instituto Dermatologico, Guadalajara, with a tentative diagnosis of leprosy.

Examination at the Instituto revealed many areas of anesthesia and hypesthesia on the macular lesions, anesthesia of the lateral margins of the feet, and alopecia of the lateral margin of the left eyebrow. The ulnar and greater auricular nerves were enlarged. Other symptoms were rhinitis, a chronic dry cough, and occasional temperature elevations to 39°C. Laboratory examinations revealed a white cell count of 14,000 per cmm, and ESR of 65. Many acid-fast bacilli and globi were seen in skin biopsies and in skin and nasal scrapings.

Epidemiological Data. The patient had always lived in small farming communities in the state of Nayarit, Mexico; he was born in the town of Ruiz. In 1962 he lived in Santiago Ixcuintla, a village of 645 people, located 20 miles from the Pacific Ocean. Santiago is in warm, mountainous dry country, 85 miles north of the popular seacoast resort city of Puerto Vallarta, and 150 miles northwest of Guadalajara.

His family group, consisting of his father, mother, and a brother, lived in an adobe house with one large room; the patient slept in a single bed. Two other brothers and a sister were married and lived elsewhere. None of the members of the immediate family was known to have had any serious illness. However, an aged uncle, with whom the patient had never lived, was described as having "claw hands," and as being chronically ill.

The patient's home had no electricity or running water, but did have a septic tank for waste disposal. The family rented this house for 35 pesos ($2.80) per month. The combined income of the patient, his father, and the brother who lived at home totalled approximately 30–40 pesos per day. The patient could read and write well and had been formally educated through the third grade.

Hospitalization at the Clinical Center (Fig. 67). The patient was observed during Study Period I, which lasted for three and one-half months. During this time, the natural periodicity of his febrile reactions became apparent. Regular examinations were made of his nasal and cutaneous scrapings, which contained many acid-fast bacilli.

Other studies revealed normal skeletal muscular strength, a sensory deficit of 27 percent of the body surface, and normal endocrine and seminal functions. His serum globulins and gamma globulins were slightly elevated; he showed a false positive Kolmer flocculation test. X-rays of the chest and skeleton were normal, and seminal vesiculogram was normal. Radiologic examination of the upper gastrointestinal tract demonstrated slight splenomegaly and outlined several *ascaris* worms in the small bowel (Fig. 66).

Leprosy bacilli were recovered in large numbers from the lymph nodes, testicles (Fig. 68), liver (Figs. 69 and 70), sputum, gastric aspirate and spermatic fascia, and in lesser numbers from the bone marrow, breast tissue and nipple discharge during an episode of acute gynecomastia. The response to intradermal lepromin was "negative."

Every four to five weeks the patient developed an acute febrile "reaction" during which he exhibited many erythema nodosum lesions, a decrease in red cell count, hematocrit and hemoglobin, and a rise in erythrocyte sedimentation rate. His body weight fell during each of these reactions. As the reactions subsided, all of the parameters which had become abnormal returned simultaneously to normal; this was associated with a rapid rise in the reticulocyte count. Each of the reactions was approximately equal in intensity with the exception of the one preceding the major surgical biopsy procedure. This reaction was less severe than previous or subsequent ones. A summary of the periodic reactions is presented in Table 16.

Cr^{51} labeling studies (Fig. 71) performed during two of his reactions demonstrated normal red cell survival, normal total blood volume, and a decreased total body red cell mass at the time of maximum anemia. On each occasion, the development of anemia was too rapid to be ascribed solely to diminished red cell formation. Water retention was ruled out as the cause of his anemia, since his total blood volume remained normal and his body weight *decreased* during the reactions. Blood loss was ruled out as a result of appropriate studies of urine and feces.

It therefore appeared that the early portion of the reaction was associated with some degree of increased hemolysis, but that this increased hemolytic activity was not a constant phenomenon. The mechanism and timing of the hemolysis was not measurable by any other studies; serum bilirubin, urobilinogen excretion, Coombs' tests and osmotic fragility measurements were normal on the occasions when they were performed. In the two most severe episodes of anemia and fever, the hematocrit fell from 38 to 29 and from 37 to 25, respectively. Recovery from anemia was associated with elevations in reticulocyte count up to 5.0 percent.

It was concluded that the anemic episodes probably represented periods of impairment of red cell formation coincident with a slightly increased rate of red cell destruction. The mechanism of the periodicity of this phenomenon, however, is still unexplained.

In Study Period II, which lasted three months, the patient was begun on small doses of DDS that were increased gradually and somewhat irregularly (because of the erythema nodosum reactions) to 100 mg per day. He was also treated with the experimental antileprosy drug, Geigy B-663. During this period he continued to experience febrile "reactions." At the end of Study Period II, however, he showed fewer leprosy bacilli in his skin and nasal scrapings, and improvement in cutaneous sensation. At this time his body weight and hematocrit were at their highest, and the ESR at its lowest, of any observations made during his entire hospitalization. In the course of Period II, also, his intestinal parasites (Table 15) disappeared spontaneously.

The patient continued to improve during the next two years with therapy utilizing DDS and B-663, as described in the report by Williams, et al. (1965).

The patient impressed the staff as a cheerful extrovert who bore the misfortune of his disease with no apparent resentment. Except for occasional malaise prior to therapy, he was consistently active and jovial. His response to chemotherapy was prompt and gratifying, and his chances for full rehabilitation seemed good.

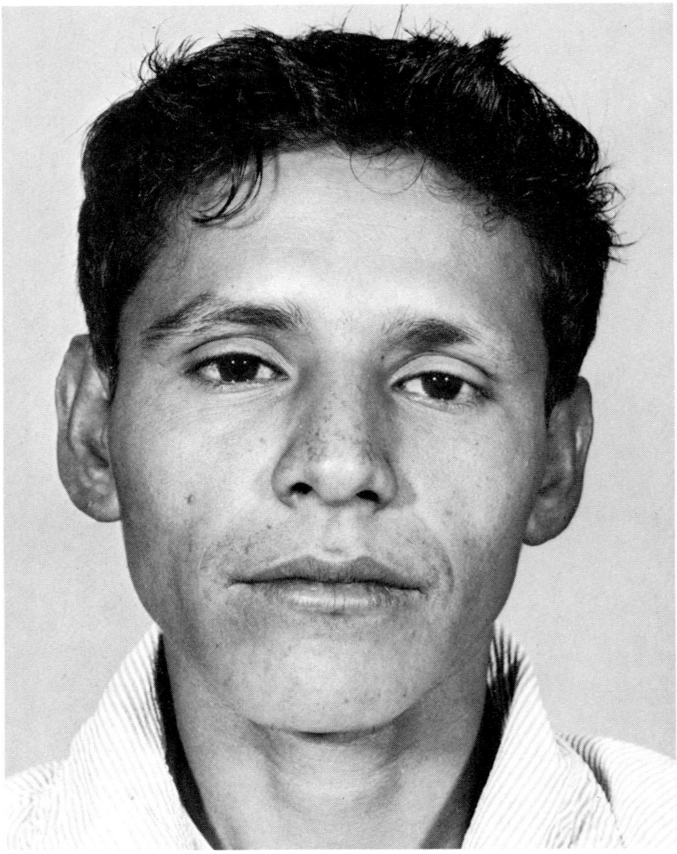

Fig. 61. A 23-year-old man: recurrent erythema nodosum episodes, chronic dermatitis of left eyebrow and both earlobes. Earlobes show induration, hyperpigmentation, tiny nodularities. (Pt. 4)

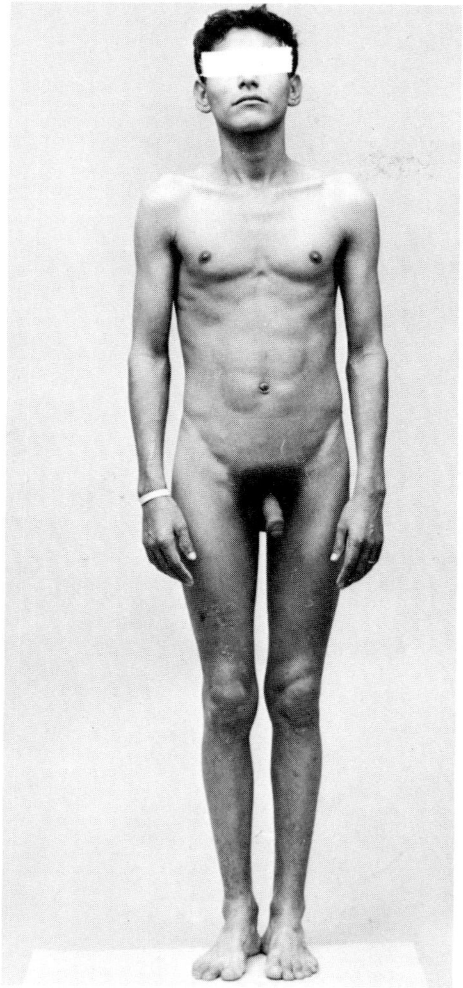

Fig. 62. Recurrent episodes of erythema nodosum have left indurated, maculopapular, hyperpigmented, anesthetic lesions of legs, forearms. Muscular development, genitalia, secondary sex characteristics, and stature, normal. (Pt. 4)

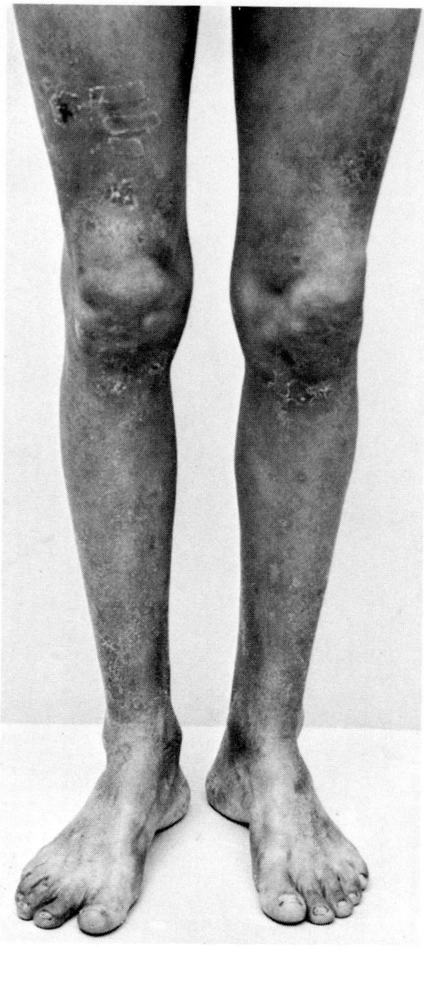

Fig. 63. Chronic lesions of erythema nodosum on legs. Histologically, many acid-fast bacilli throughout dermis and subcutaneous tissues. Widespread distal hypesthesia; no muscular atrophy apparent. (Pt. 4)

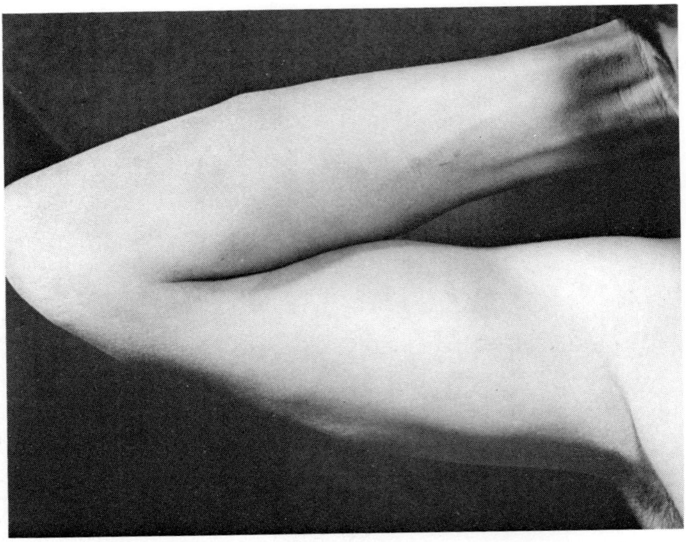

Fig. 64. Active erythema nodosum lesions on forearms and arm: painful, tender for three to four days. When fever subsided, nodules disappeared, skin normal. (Pt. 4)

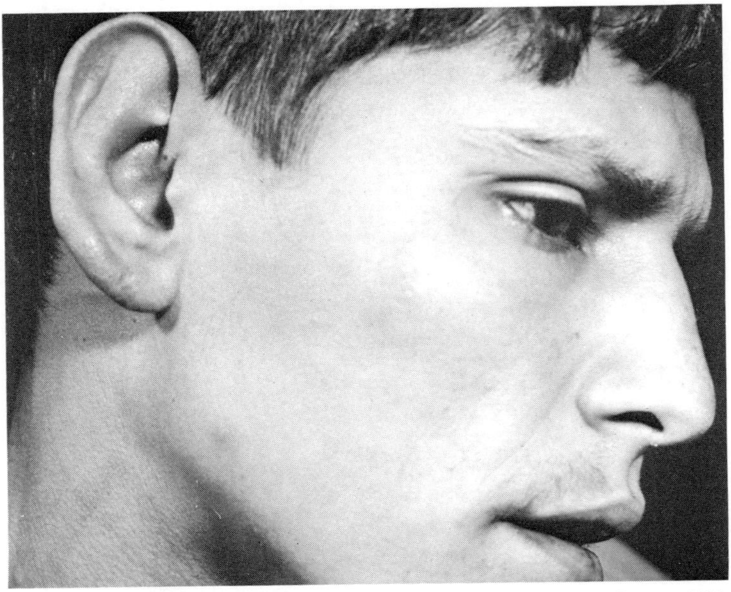

Fig. 65. Erythema nodosum lesions of face at angle of mandible, simulating a furuncle. Tiny chronic nodularities on earlobe are visible. Not apparent in photograph is diffuse erythema of malar eminence accompanying febrile reaction. Mouth is open because of rhinitis accompanying reaction. (Pt. 4)

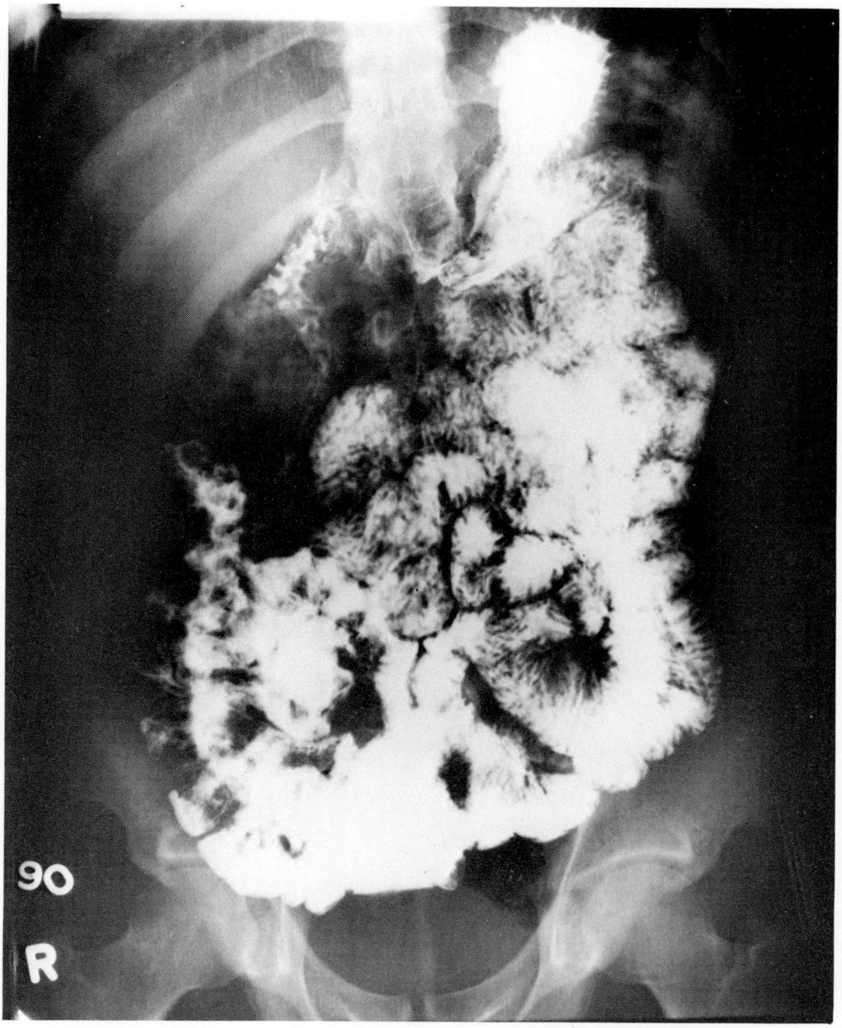

Fig. 66. X-ray, gastrointestinal. GI series shows *Ascaris lumbricoides* outlined in small bowel, left lower quadrant. Indentations of barium column by liver and spleen do not reveal significant enlargement of these organs. Compare patient 1, Fig. 11. (Pt. 4)

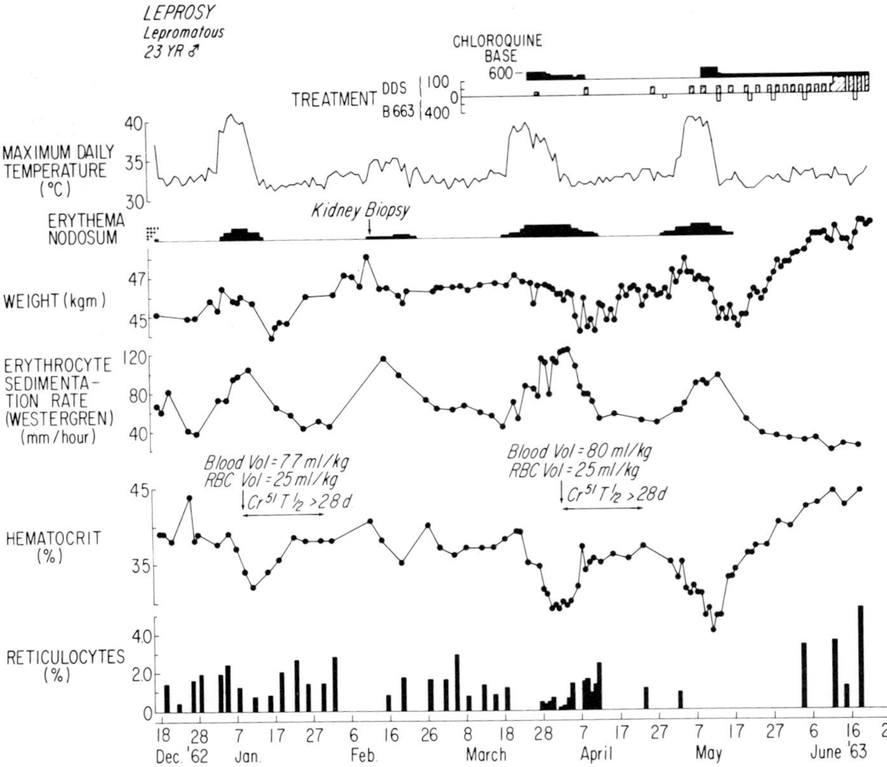

Fig. 67. Clinical Course Chart. Weight decreased with each monthly episode of fever and erythema nodosum until DDS and B663 therapy started. Sedimentation rate was markedly elevated with each reaction, declined during therapy. Periodic episodes of anemia were apparently of complex origin. (Pt. 4)

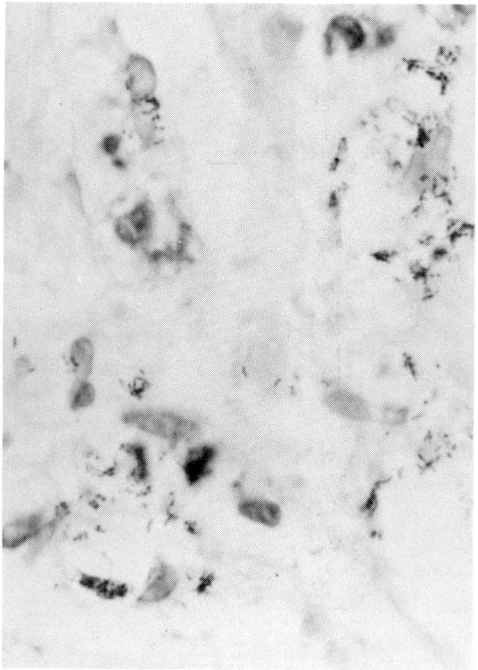

Fig. 68. Photomicrograph, testicle. Many acid-fast bacilli in interstitial areas and within tubules; no bacilli in semen. Testicles were slightly enlarged and firm but within normal limits. No gross indication of testicular infection; spermatogenesis normal. Fite stain, 1010X. (Pt. 4)

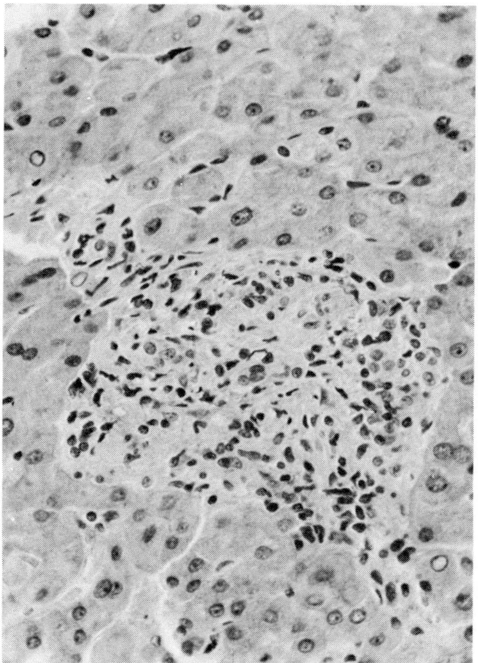

Fig. 69. Photomicrograph, liver. This illustration gives no indication of massive infiltration by acid-fast bacilli in hepatic granulomas. Bacterial stain required (see Fig. 70). Compare patient 2, Fig. 37, showing no acid-fast bacilli. H & E stain, 250X. (Pt. 4)

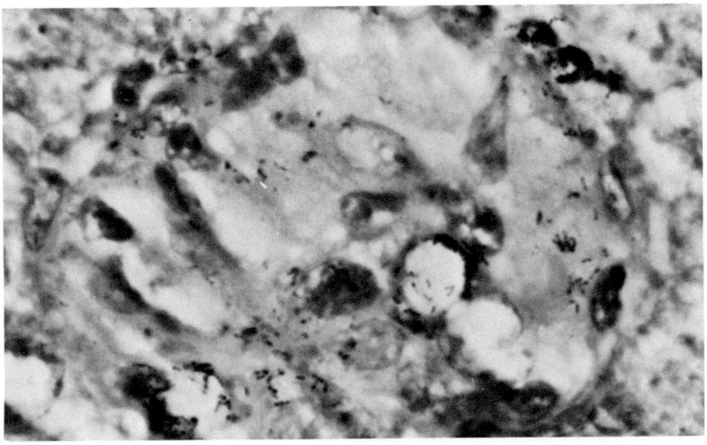

Fig. 70. Photomicrograph, liver. Hepatic granuloma, showing many acid-fast bacilli in macrophages with cytoplasmic vacuoles. Few organisms seen in liver cells adjacent to granuloma. Fite stain, 1010X. (Pt. 4)

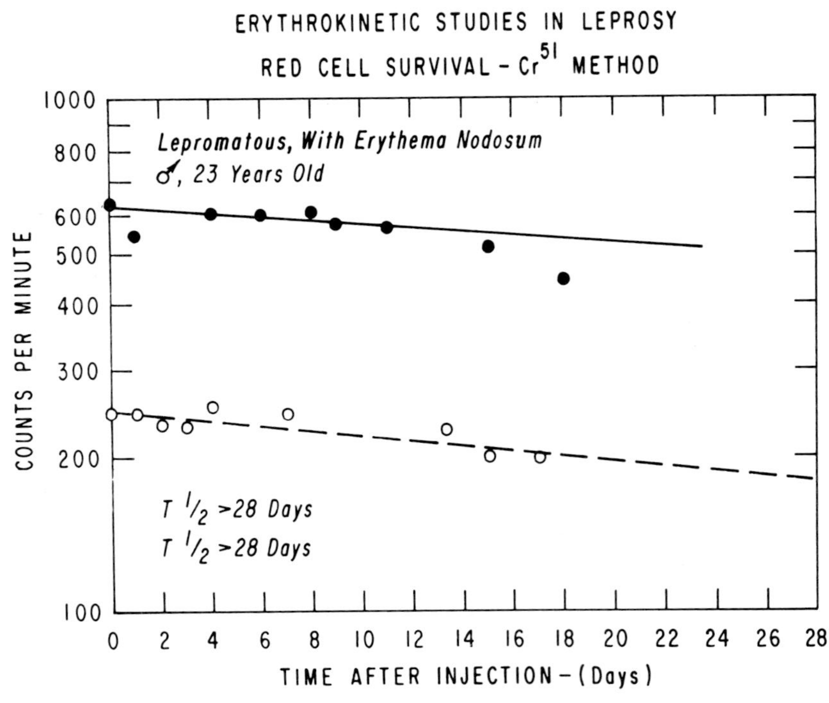

Fig. 71. Red cell survival normal, as measured by Cr^{51} RBC T½. Red cell survival studies were carried out at periods of maximum anemia, as recorded in Fig. 67. (Pt.4)

PATIENT 5

A 25-Year-Old Male of Mestizo Extraction

Symptomatic from leprous infection in many areas of his body, frightened and psychologically depressed (Figs. 72–74). Tentative Diagnosis: Leprosy, lepromatous, or possibly dimorphous. Final Diagnosis: Lepromatous leprosy, nodular type.

History. Approximately four years prior to admission, the patient noticed the gradual onset of anesthesia of the extremities, dryness of the skin, and fissures on his heels. He had previously noticed nodules on his face and chest, and a large, irregular, raised hyperchromic area on the upper portion of his face. His nose and ears became enlarged and he developed severe malaise, short thick fingers and a poor grasp. Recurrent trauma to his fingers, and blisters on his feet had resulted in scarring and chronic ulceration.

He was concerned about this progressive disease, which he assumed was "contagious," and had consequently avoided the company of his friends for approximately two years. He sought the advice of a local irregular practitioner, who treated him with herbs and put him in a closed dark, hot room for 40 days. This "treatment" took all of his money and left him feeling extremely weak. He then decided to come to the city and ask for medical assistance. He feared that he had leprosy, and had been told by his friends that lepers were executed by being boiled in oil.

At the Instituto Dermatologica in Guadalajara acid-fast bacilli were found on cutaneous scrapings. The patient was observed at that time to have enlargement of ulnar, radial, popliteal and tibial nerves.

Epidemiological Data. The patient had lived all his life in Ocotlan, Jalisco, 40 miles southeast of Guadalajara. Ocotlan is a rural community (population 17,000) which specializes in the manufacture of pottery. The town is situated a few miles from Mexico's largest lake, Lake Chapala, and is a popular spot for fishermen and tourists.

The patient lived in a two-room adobe cottage with his mother; each slept in a separate room. This house had a dirt floor, no electricity or water, and no toilet facilities. The patient's three married sisters lived in an adjacent house.

One of the patient's sisters was under treatment for "red spots" and was believed to have leprosy. The patient's father died five years previously, of "kidney disease." Four years previously the patient's wife left him, taking their newborn daughter with her. A previous child had died in infancy and nothing was known about the health of the patient's wife or his daughter. This story was strongly reminiscent of the family of the legendary Pedro Martinez, who was Oscar Lewis' (1964) prototype of a Mexican peasant.

The patient came to the Instituto Dermatologico with a person who had been a "friend" for many years, and who was known to have leprosy. His friend occasionally appeared at the Instituto to receive therapy.

Hospitalization at the Clinical Center (Fig. 75). The three-month period of observation was designated Study Period I. During this time he received symptomatic therapy and hygienic care for the ulcerations and calluses of his extremities. Many acid-fast bacilli, including globi, were found in skin and nasal scrapings (Figs. 76 and 77). These organisms were also seen in biopsies of the liver, lymph nodes (Fig. 78), and testicles (Figs. 79 and 80). Acid-fast bacilli were present in gastric aspirate and in urethral discharge obtained after prostatic massage. Acid-fast bacilli were also found in bone marrow, conjunctival scrapings and in the renal biopsy specimen (Fig. 81). No giant cells or granulomas were found in any of the biopsies.

There was considerable inflammation and decreased spermatogenesis in the testicle, and necrotic areas filled with acid-fast bacilli were observed in the liver. The skin showed many types of involvement by leprosy. Massive numbers of leprosy bacilli were present in the prepuce removed at circumcision. However, no organisms were seen in biopsies of pubic and axillary skin. A female *Ascaris lumbricoides* worm recovered from feces after "Antepar" therapy showed red-shaped acid-fast structures in the ovaries similar to the bacilli in the liver biopsy. Acid-fast structures were not present in a control specimen of *A. lumbricoides* obtained from a young North Carolina boy who did not have leprosy.

Patient 5 had sensory abnormalities of 50 percent of his body surface although skeletal muscular strength was normal. Total serum globulin and gamma globulin concentrations were elevated; he had a high erythrocyte sedimentation rate. Although his production of 17OH corticosteroids was normal, his 17-ketosteroid production was moderately depressed, consistent with partial testicular destruction. A seminal vesiculogram showed an obstructed outflow bilaterally (Fig. 82).

X-rays of the hands revealed resorption of the digital tufts and monoarticular septic arthritis (Fig. 83). His response to intradermal lepromin was "negative" when compared with the "positive" response evoked by injection of the same material in a normal person (Fig. 85). Red blood cell survival was normal (Fig. 84), based on Cr^{51} studies.

Subsequently, this patient received B-663 for one year, and was bacteriologically improved. But he developed severe pigmentation of the nodular lesions, malaise, and weight loss, and was thought to be suffering from drug toxicity. In 1965 sputum specimens revealed *Mycobacterium tuberculosis* for the first time. Treatment with isoniazid (INH) and para-aminosalicylic acid (PAS) was instituted, and the patient again improved. The details of therapy with B-663 and the subsequent course are fully described in Williams, et al. (1965).

Patient 5 was a large, dark-skinned man with moderately severe leonine facies. Since this physiognomy was uncommon in the United States, he was not recognized as a person with leprosy in casual contacts with laymen. In Mexico, on the other hand, he had been fearful of being shunned as a "Lazarino" — a leper. He came to the Clinical Center frightened and depressed, and found it difficult to adjust to the reality of his disease and to his hospitalization.

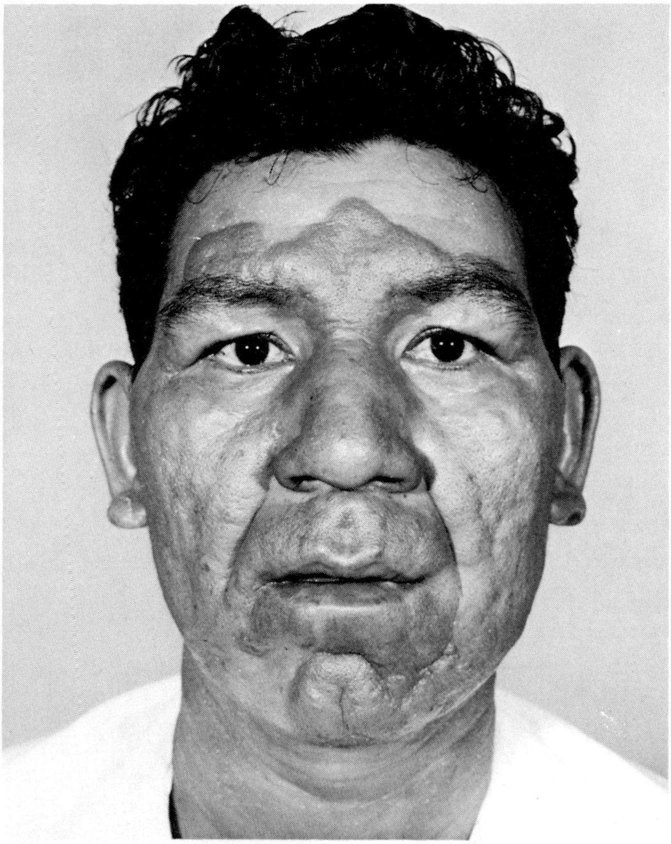

Fig. 72. A 25-year-old man: indurated skin, decreased sensitivity to pin prick and touch over entire lower face and ears. Skin hyperpigmented, hyperkeratotic; earlobes enlarged, nodular. Mouth ajar because of rhinitis. Perspiration on forehead and neck; lower face does not perspire due to destruction of peripheral nerves to sweat glands. (Pt. 5)

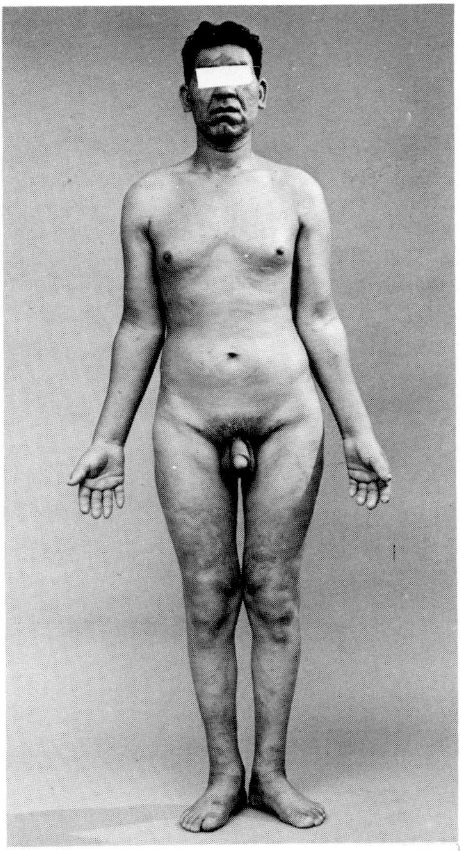

Fig. 73. Body vitrually hairless. Much of skin surface consists of irregular, raised hyperchromic macules. Breasts enlarged; fingers and toes short, thick, ulcerated at tips. (Pt. 5)

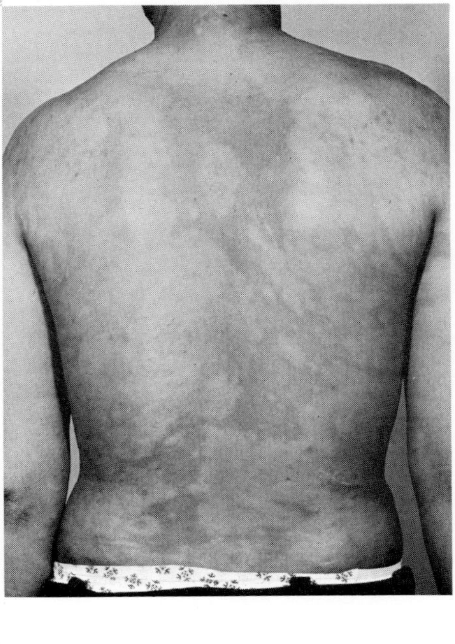

Fig. 74. Close-up view, maculopapular hyperchromic rash, with central hypochromicity. Well-healed right flank renal biopsy incision is visible. Back has many areas of hypesthesia, other areas of cutaneous tenderness. (Pt. 5)

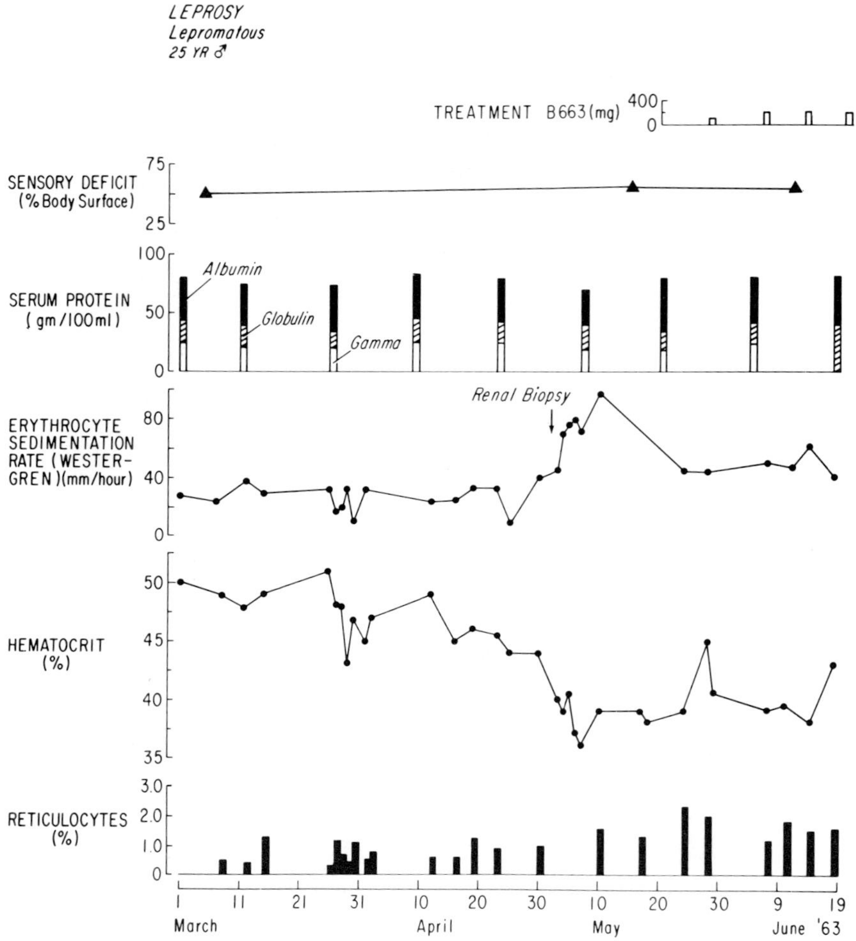

Fig. 75. Clinical Course Chart. Initial three-month stability but persistent decline in hematocrit; sedimentation rate chronically elevated, became markedly elevated following renal biopsy—this attributed mainly to nonspecific inflammatory factors. (Pt. 5)

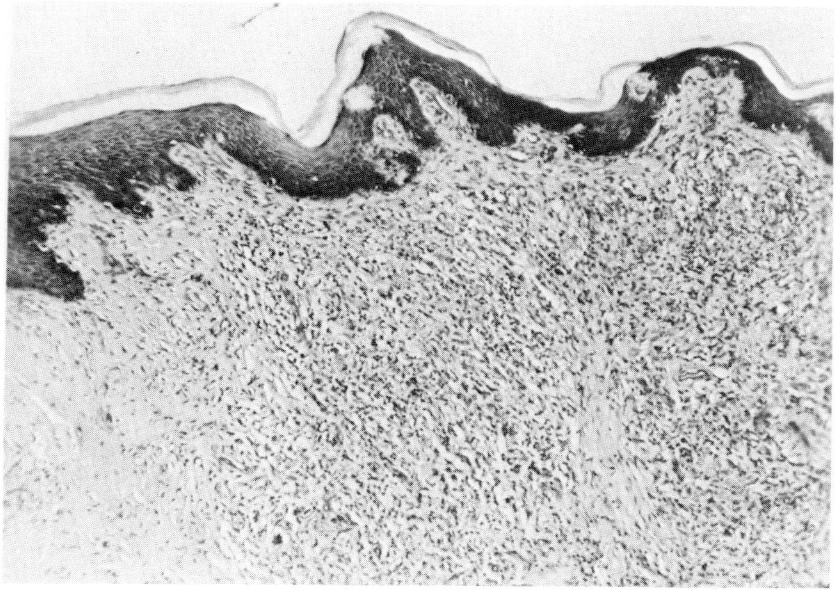

Fig. 76. Photomicrograph, foreskin. Lepromatous balanoposthitis. Mononuclear cells contain myriads of acid-fast bacilli. Fite stain, 70X. (Pt. 5)

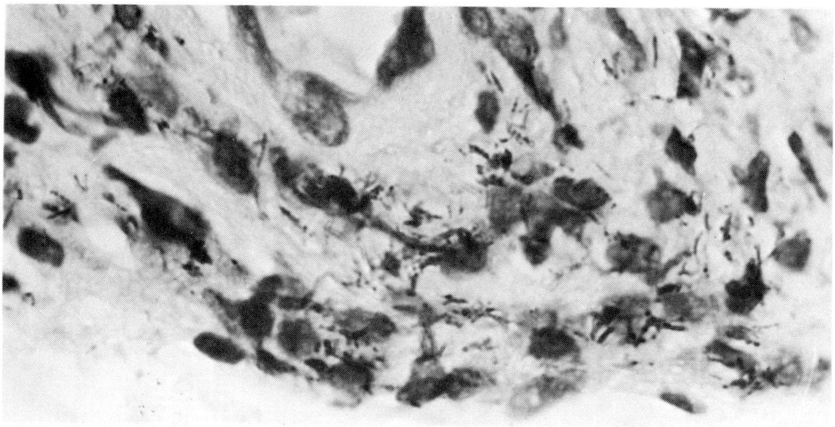

Fig. 77. Photomicrograph, foreskin; a closer view of specimen in Fig. 76. Intense lepromatous perivasculitis. Density of organisms in foreskin appeared to be greater than in any other cutaneous area. Fite stain, 939X. (Pt. 5)

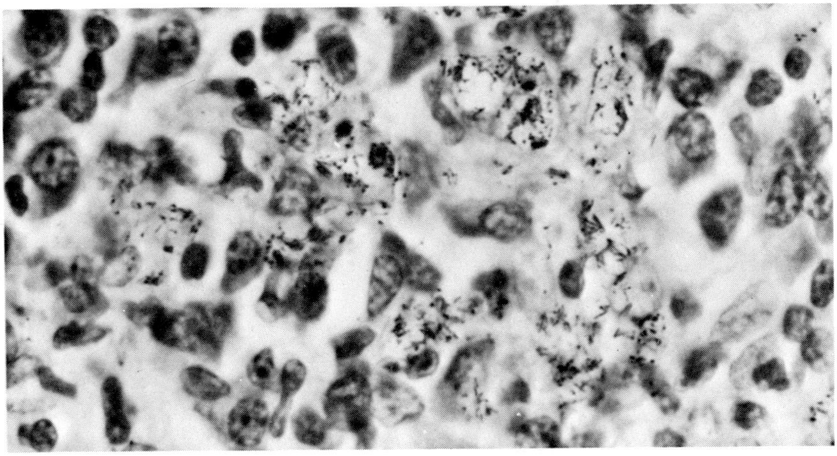

Fig. 78. Photomicrograph, inguinal lymph node. Enlarged, soft, non-tender. Contained large numbers of acid-fast bacilli. Granularity more apparent than in skin, testicle (Fig. 80) and glomerulus (Fig. 81). Compare patient 3, Fig. 49; patient 4, Fig. 70; patient 1, Figs. 16 and 18. Fite stain, 939X. (Pt. 5)

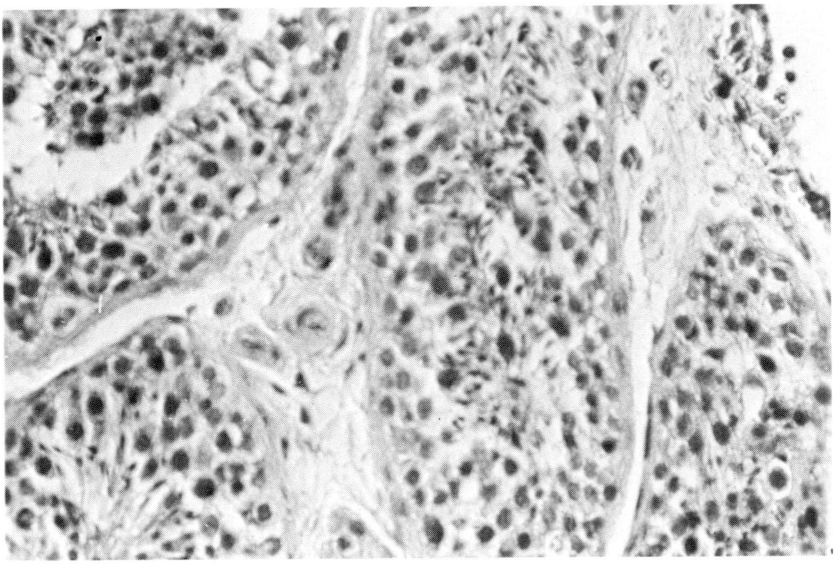

Fig. 79. Photomicrograph, testicle. Normal architecture and spermatogenesis. Gross examination revealed no definite pathologic features. Under higher magnification (Fig. 80) same area shows interstitial lepromatous infiltration. H & E stain, 288X. (Pt. 5)

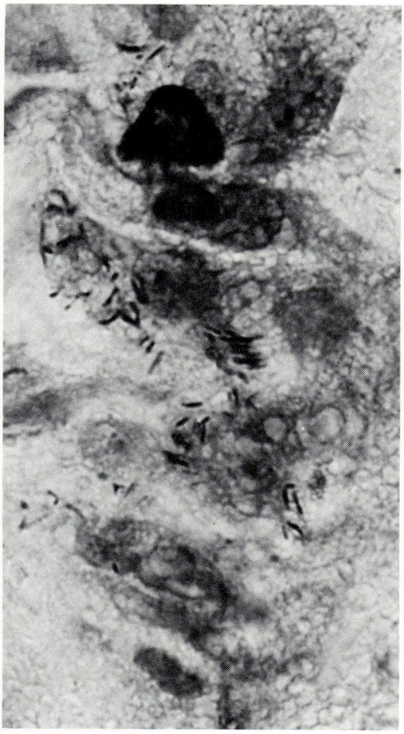

Fig. 80. Photomicrograph, testicle. Acid-fast bacilli in globi and as isolated organisms, in interstitial areas. In other areas, organisms seen within seminiferous tubules. Fite stain, 1010X. (Pt. 5)

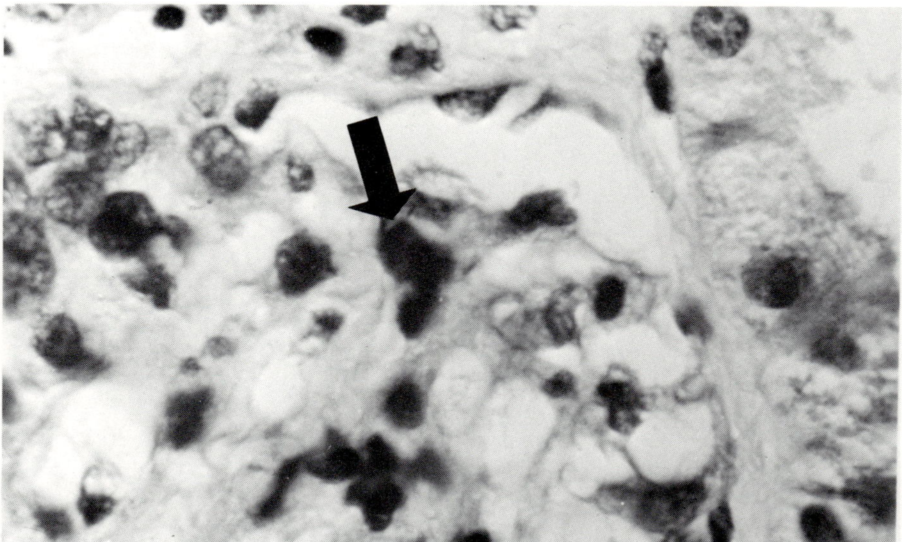

Fig. 81. Photomicrograph, kidney. Several acid-fast bacilli in a capillary of the glomerulus, seen here with Fite stain, 1010X. (Pt. 5)

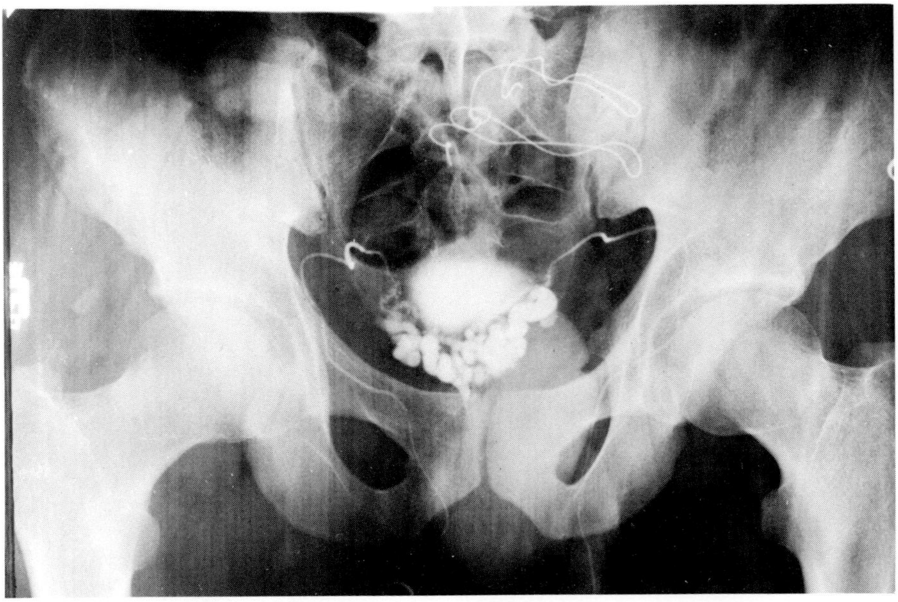

Fig. 82. X-ray, seminal vesiculogram. Partial obstruction of seminal vesicles, as in patients 2 and 4. Normal seminal vesiculograms observed in patients 1 and 3, no obstructive pattern in patient 1. Infertility in leprosy patients probably due to lepromatous orchitis. (Pt. 5)

Fig. 83. X-ray, hands. Osteomyelitis, loss of portions of terminal phalanges of seven digits. Osteitis in right thumb. Multiple superficial erosions and infections in soft tissues especially at finger tips, joints. (Pt. 5)

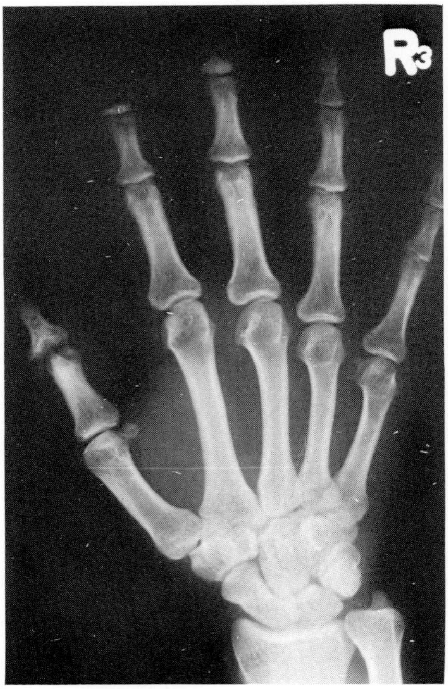

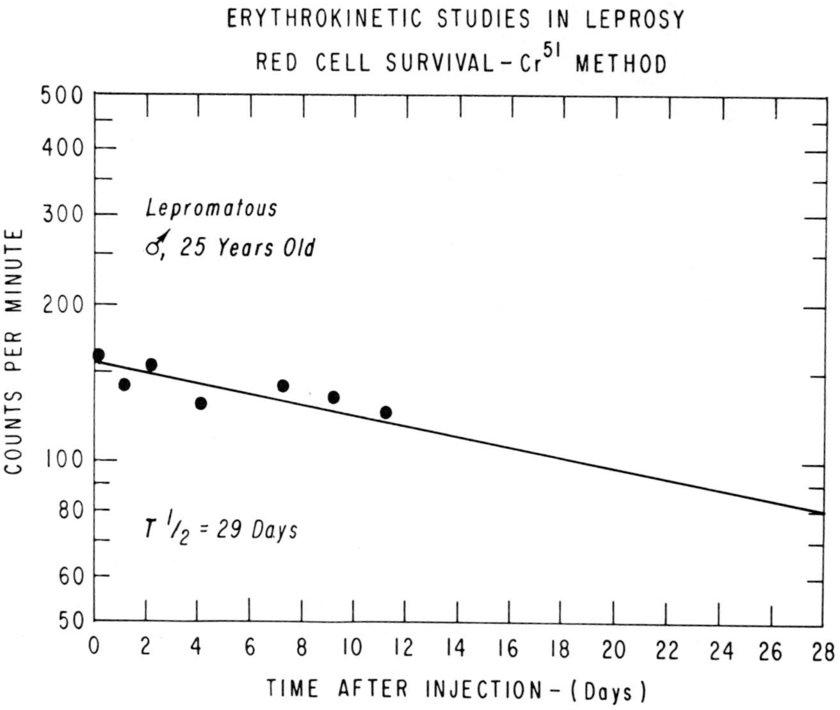
ERYTHROKINETIC STUDIES IN LEPROSY
RED CELL SURVIVAL - Cr51 METHOD
COUNTS PER MINUTE
500
400
300
200
100
80
60
50
Lepromatous
♂, 25 Years Old
T 1/2 = 29 Days
0
2
4
6
8
10
12
14
16
18
20
22
24
26
28
TIME AFTER INJECTION - (Days)

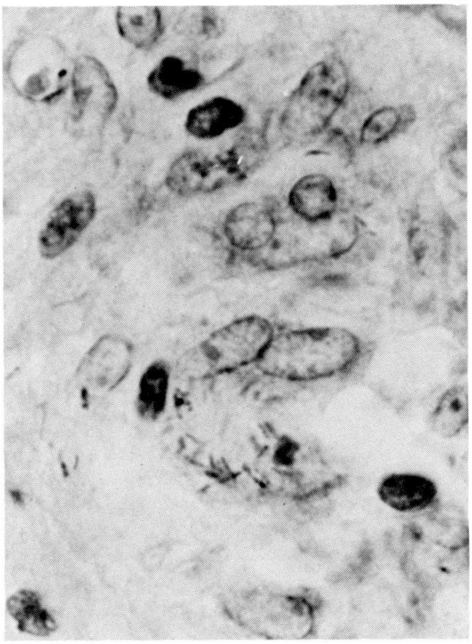

Fig. 85. Photomicrograph, lepromin skin test in *normal* person. A "positive" response in normal person, biopsied 21 days after intradermal injection of 0.1 ml of lepromin. Intense inflammatory reaction observed grossly; on microscopic examinations, injected microorganisms engulfed in macrophages. Cellular response predominantly macrophages and lymphocytes; occasional giant cells observed. Fite stain, 1010X.

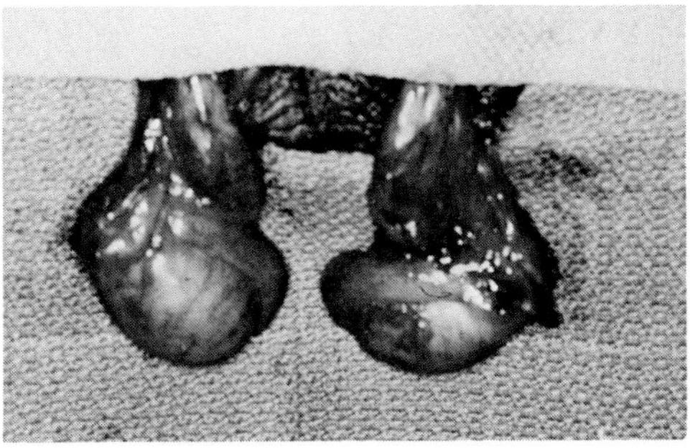

Fig. 86. Operating room photograph, testicles of patient 1. Atrophy and total destruction of spermatogenesis, associated with severe lepromatous orchitis. Eunuchoid level of urinary chorionic gonadotrophin. 4.0 × 2.0 cm.

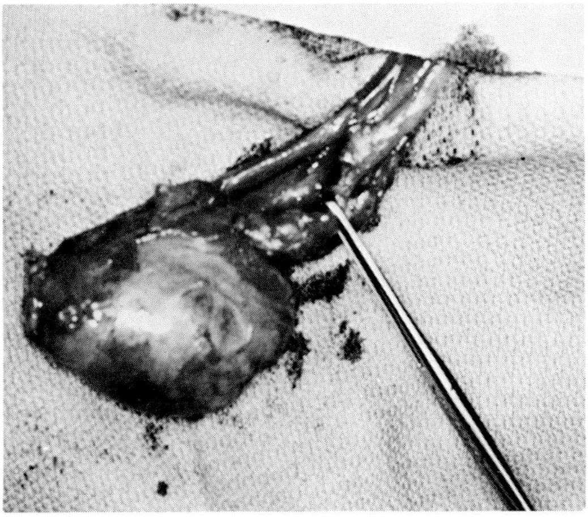

Fig. 87. Operating room photograph, testicles of patient 2. Hypertrophy due to fibrosis, associated with tubular atrophy and decrease in spermatogenesis. No acid-fast bacilli present, but external spermatic nerve (at tip of pointer) was 5 mm in diameter, contained granulomas with giant cells. 6.0 × 4.5 cm.

SERUM ELECTROPHORESIS IN LEPROSY
(PRIOR TO THERAPY)

	Total Protein	Albumin	α_1	α_2	β	γ
NORMAL	6.7-8.2 gm%	53-68%	2-6%	5-13%	8-16%	9-21%

LEPROMATOUS (DIFFUSE)
♂17 Years
04-22-53

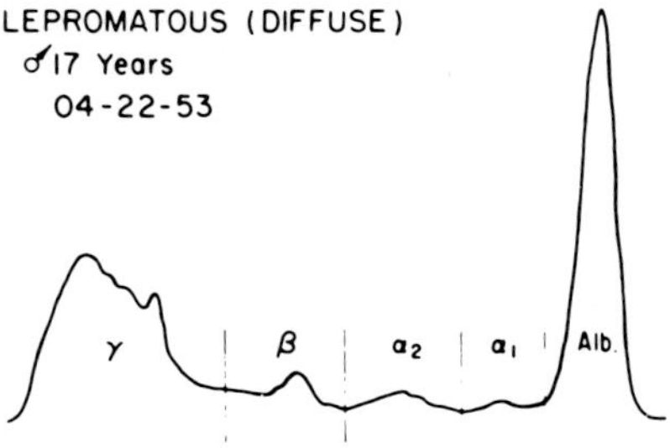

Total Protein	Albumin	α_1	α_2	β	γ
9.5	29.6	2.6	4.5	7.8	55.5

INDETERMINATE → LEPROMATOUS
♂14 Years
04-22-55

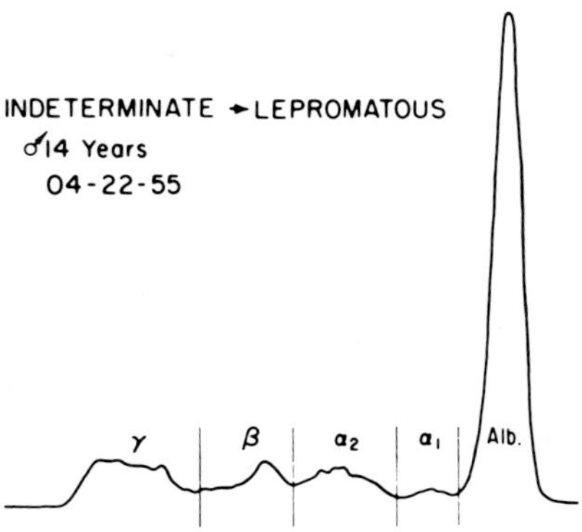

Total Protein	Albumin	α_1	α_2	β	γ
8.0	56.0	2.6	12.1	10.3	19.0

DIMORPHOUS → TUBERCULOID
♂27 Years
04-22-54

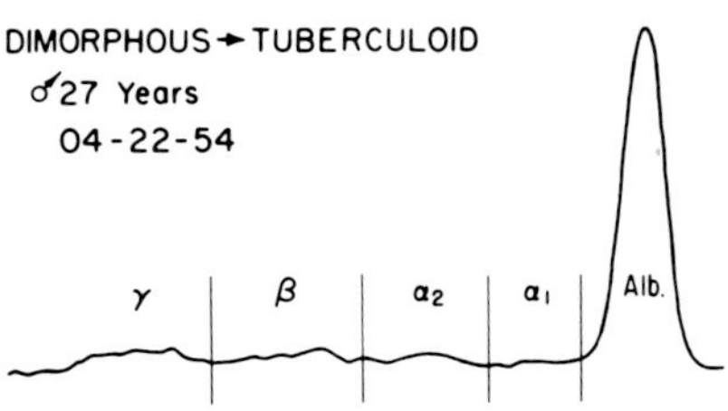

Total Protein	Albumin	α_1	α_2	β	γ
7.1	64.5	3.2	8.1	12.9	11.3

Fig. 88. Serum protein electrophoresis in leprosy (prior to therapy). Paper electrophoresis of serum from patient 1 revealed elevation in total serum proteins, due to elevation in gamma globulin concentration. No specific abnormalities observed in patients 2 and 3. Studies were performed in NIH Clinical Chemistry Laboratory under supervision of Dr. Ernest Cotlove.

SERUM IMMUNOELECTROPHORESIS IN LEPROSY
(*Prior to therapy*)

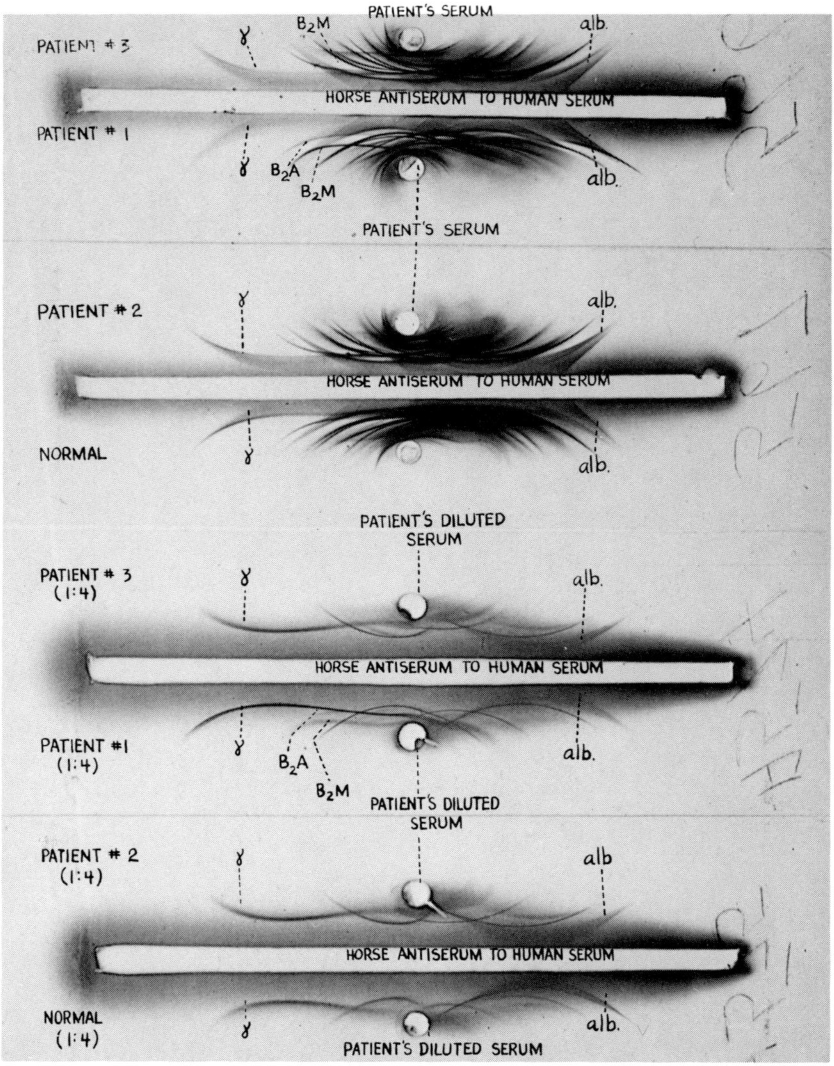

Fig. 89. Serum immunoelectrophoresis in leprosy (prior to therapy). An elevated concentration of γ (IgG), B_2M (IgM) and B_2A (IgA) proteins observed in patient 1, elevated concentration of B_2M (IgM) in patient 3. Labelling of illustration by author is based upon Kabat, E. A., and Mayer, M. M., *Experimental Immunochemistry*, 2nd Ed., 1961, p. 648.

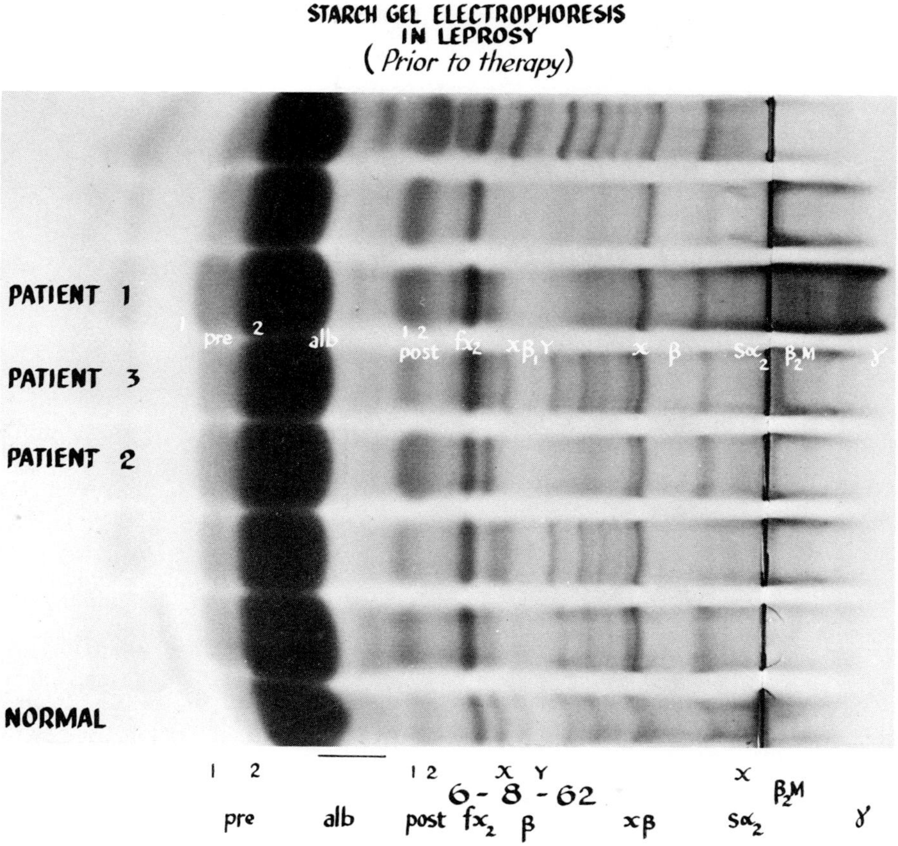

Fig. 90. Starch gel electrophoresis of serum in leprosy (prior to therapy). A remarkably dense globulin band was seen in the serum of patient 1. Variation in lines in "$\alpha\beta$" area between $F\alpha_2$ and $S\alpha_2$ in the three patients probably due to genetic differences in haptoglobins. Electrophoreses were performed by Drs. Sheldon Wolff, Howard Goodman, John Fahey, and José Uriel.

DISCUSSION

"You have to move, live, breathe, see, hear, in the midst of millions of people, not daring to touch one of them, afraid to speak lest they become friendly—avoiding—avoiding—eternally avoiding."

Perry Burgess, *Who Walk Alone*

I. THE SKIN

Abnormalities of the Skin (Table 2)

An abnormality of the skin is usually the first sign of infection with leprosy; in most cases it is skin disease which brings the patient with leprosy to a doctor. References to leprosy in history and literature are usually made in terms of abnormalities of the skin. The "lepra" or "scaly" disease described by Hippocrates, and the "leprous" disease of King Uzziah's forehead (2 Chron. 26:12–23) may or may not have been the disease caused by the bacillus described by Hansen in 1874.

Medieval laymen and physicians were able to distinguish acute contagious diseases, such as plague, from the chronic diseases which they called leprosy. But the fungal skin diseases, psoriasis, and other noncontagious dermatologic disorders were undoubtedly confused with leprosy. In particular, patients with alopecia areata and vitiligo must have been subject to the special "burial services" and social exclusions customary for lepers in the Middle Ages.*

Hansen's discovery of *M. leprae*, and the discovery of *M. tuberculosis* by Koch (1882) did not immediately clarify the nature of these mycobacterial diseases. As late as 1906 Sir Jonathan Hutchinson proclaimed that leprosy was caused by the ingestion of rotten fish. Gradually, however, leprosy was recognized as a bacterial infection. In a vivid description of a leprosy patient with alopecia, ulcerations and red nodules, Sir William Osler (1898) credited Hansen with the discovery of the cause of leprosy.

In spite of modern advances in the epidemiology and pathology of leprosy, the diagnosis is usually made only after the patient inquires about a skin lesion. The abnormality may be an anesthetic area, as in the case of the boy from Colorado, "Ned Langford," described by Burgess (1951). This young man had been inadvertently billeted with a leprous family in the Philippines and infection became apparent in him nine years later.

"Pale rose spots" were the first signs of leprosy to appear in

* The tragic history of leprosy and lepers has been reviewed by A. Weymouth. His book, *The Leper Squint* (1938), derives its name from the narrow slits in the walls of medieval churches where lepers were permitted to observe services.

"Betty Martin" (1950), who – like Burgess' patient – was destined to spend almost a lifetime in a leprosy hospital. As an adolescent "Betty Martin" lived in New Orleans, where leprosy is endemic; however, she had no known contacts with leprosy victims.

Anesthesia and nodules of leprosy first appeared in Father Damien at the age of 45 after twelve years of ministry to lepers at Molokai. He had come to the Hawaiian Islands as a young man of 24. In spite of his illness, he continued to work vigorously until his death at the age of 49. (Farrow, 1954.)

The historical and scientific importance of the skin in leprosy will become evident in this discussion. In our analysis of the information derived from the five young leprosy patients studied at the NIH Clinical Center, we give first priority to abnormalities of the skin. The system of classification of leprosy used in the NIH study was that of the Leonard Wood Memorial (Doull, 1954). This classification follows the recommendation presented to the VI International Congress of Leprosy, Madrid, 1953, except that the term "dimorphous" has been substituted for the term "borderline."

Symptoms.

All five patients were aware of disease of the skin. Because of skin lesions, two patients (1 and 5) totally avoided contact with society except for their relatives. Another patient (2) was sensitive about his changed appearance but continued to work more or less regularly as a salesman. Of the remaining two patients, one (4) appeared to have no uneasiness in social situations as a result of his appearance. This was true of the other (3) until he developed exfoliative dermatitis, atrophy of the hands, and a leonine appearance of his face, when he often felt too embarrassed to leave his hospital room.

Inspection.

Leprosy has classically been regarded as primarily an infectious disease involving the skin and peripheral nerves. As a general rule it may be said that on careful examination a patient with leprosy will usually manifest some abnormality of the surface of the skin.

The five patients in this study are no exceptions to this rule.

Induration of the skin was present in all of them, and one demonstrated areas of atrophy. Four of the patients had hypochromic macules and three also had hyperchromic macules, nodules, or nodosities, some with hypochromic centers. The earlobes were enlarged or contained tiny nodosities in four of the patients; enlargement of the nasal alae was present in three.

Alopecia was evident in three patients. Loss of the hair of the eyebrows and eyelashes was virtually complete in one of these patients and partially complete in another. It was particularly interesting that the loss of eyebrow hair in Patient 1 was not associated with loss of scalp hair, as illustrated in Fig. 5. Alopecia of macules was present in three patients, one of whom manifested hairless macules on his lower face.

Cutaneous nerve enlargement was visible upon inspection in three patients, trophic abnormalities of the soft tissue of the hands and feet in four patients, and traumatic lesions in anesthetic areas of the hands and feet in three. Erythema nodosum lesions were present in two patients; one of these had in addition an extensive exfoliative dermatitis. One patient's skin was ulcerated due apparently to thrombotic lepromatous arteritis. These ulcers, known as Lucio lesions (Latapí, 1948), may also have been caused by local trauma.

Anhidrosis of extensive areas of the body was observed in patients 1, 2 and 3, who were examined in the hot, humid controlled-environment chamber. One patient (2) demonstrated cutaneous capillary fragility in anesthetic areas. This abnormality was most obvious when the skin was observed about 30 minutes after a sensory examination, at which time each pin prick in the anesthetic areas was the center of a 2–3 mm punctate hemorrhage.

Four of the five patients experienced pain in the skin at some time during their illness. Patient 1 felt acute pain in each Lucio lesion for 36–48 hours after its onset. No further symptoms were observed as the Lucio lesions progressed to superficial necrosis and scar formation. Patient 2 reported considerable pain in his erythematous macules, but as discoloration of the macules subsided and normal sensation returned the pain disappeared. Patient 3 complained of diffuse cutaneous pain, especially severe in the erythema nodosum lesions at the time of his "reaction"; he was often troubled with insomnia because of generalized hyperalgesia. Patient 4 experienced moderate pain and hyperalgesia in his erythema nodosum lesions during the monthly episodes of fever and generalized weakness.

One patient (1) showed extreme concern about his alopecia. In the initial stages of DDS therapy he was often seen examining his eyebrows and eyelashes for a return of hair. No regrowth of hair could possibly be demonstrated, however, during his five months of therapy with DDS. In three of the other patients small areas of alopecia were noticeable on the extremities and trunk. They showed no particular concern over the loss of hair, which was not progressive during their hospitalization.

Histopathology of the Skin.

The cross-sectional skin of each patient was observed in the operating room at the time biopsy was performed; the gross appearance was usually a good indication of the severity of the histological abnormalities present. In general, the histologic features of the cutaneous lesions in the five patients confirmed the classic descriptions of Fite (1943) and Binford (1958).

Atrophy of the epidermis was grossly apparent in three of the patients (1, 2 and 3), whose skin was excessively smooth on the surface. This gross appearance, suggesting epidermal atrophy and flattening of the rete pegs, was confirmed histologically. Hyperkeratosis was grossly and microscopically apparent in the margins of the erythematous macules of patient 2, in the desquamating skin of patient 3, and in the skin of the thigh of patient 4, which was subject to recurrent erythema nodosum lesions similar to those described by Canizares (1962).*

In two of the patients (1 and 5) the flank incision revealed thickening of the skin due to confluent inflammation infiltrating and extending into the subcutaneous tissues. The skin in these areas was leathery in texture and difficult to suture. Sensation in the flank skin was normal, but the cutaneous nerves were greatly enlarged and contained masses of acid-fast bacilli.

In one other patient (4) a moderate degree of subcutaneous

* Perivascular infiltration with acute and chronic inflammatory cells is a prominent feature of erythema nodosum leprosum (ENL). The similarity of ENL to the Arthus phenomenon was recently pointed out by Wemambu, et al. (1969). They demonstrated deposits of immunoglobulin, complement and mycobacterial antigens in the areas of polymorphonuclear leukocyte infiltration in ENL, which were similar to perivascular immune complexes in laboratory animals with the Arthus phenomenon.

extension of inflammatory cells was present. The foreskin specimen which was obtained at circumcision in patient 5 was markedly indurated, but did not appear grossly different from more prosaic forms of balanoposthitis. However, the specimen showed histologically that extensive collections of leprosy bacilli were present in large foamy macrophages (Virchow's cells).

In general, the structures which showed the most extensive abnormalities in biopsies of normal-appearing skin (such as the first biopsy specimens of patient 3) were the cutaneous nerves. In the biopsies of patient 2, organisms could be found *only* in dermal nerves and granulomas. Collections of inflammatory cells containing bacilli were demonstrated widely throughout the dermis, but most prominently around blood vessels, dermal appendages (hair follicles, sweat glands, and sebaceous glands), and nerves. Dense accumulations of bacilli were present in Schwann cells, or along nerve fibers, or immediately within the perineurium — in short, throughout the peripheral nerves.

Bacilli were rarely seen in the epidermis, except in patient 1, where necrotic epidermis containing organisms was present overlying the arterial thrombosis in a Lucio lesion. The cutaneous arteries of the legs in this patient had greatly thickened muscular walls, containing intramural lymphocytes, bacilli, and globi.

Acid-fast bacilli were often seen intraluminally in the endothelial cells of blood vessels (arteries, veins, capillaries and lymphatics). Biopsy of a tender, hypesthetic hyperchromic macule in patient 2 revealed granulomatous arteritis without acid-fast bacilli. The arterial walls were thickened and contained Langhans giant cells.

The study of biopsies obtained simultaneously from a number of skin sites on each patient was especially instructive. The distribution of acid-fast bacilli in the deep viscera (lymphatics, liver, testicles, etc.) of each patient had been well documented: in all except patient 2 organisms had been found to be widely distributed. It was therefore of interest to discover that even in patients with extensive deep involvement by *M. leprae* (Table 4) only rarely were acid-fast bacilli present in areas of normal hair growth — the scalp, axilla, and pubis. In patient 1 the only cutaneous area which was completely free of bacilli was the dense collagenous tissue in the bed of a Lucio lesion scar.

The specimens obtained from patient 5 showed a greater

degree of granularity of the leprosy bacilli than did those of the other four patients. However, in none of the patients were differences apparent in the staining qualities of organisms recovered from the skin as compared to those recovered from the lymph nodes, liver, kidneys, blood stream, testicles, or elsewhere. The number of bacilli in skin scrapings and in skin biopsies decreased in patients 2 and 3 during their hospitalization. This quantitative change could not be correlated, however, with a qualitative alteration in the appearance of the bacilli or with the appearance of any extracellular acid-fast material in these biopsies.

The earlobes were enlarged in four of the patients. Earlobe biopsies of three of these patients revealed an extensive network of dermal capillaries; the earlobes of patients 4 and 5 contained many acid-fast bacilli.

Lepromin Tests, Evolution and Histology.

Lepromin skin tests were performed in three normal volunteers, and in three leprosy patients. The lepromin used was designated "integral lepromin"; it was a glycerine suspension of ground lepromas, sterilized by tyndallization. It had been prepared three years previously, in 1959, and was supplied by the Centro Dermatologico Pascua. A "positive" reaction was defined as a nodule at least 5 mm in diameter present 21 days after injection.

All three normal volunteers showed "positive" reactions to 0.1 ml injected intradermally. Twenty-four hours after injection, nodules developed (the Fernandez reaction) which were 10–15 mm in diameter, erythematous and intensely pruritic. These nodules subsided in one week. The nodules *reappeared* after another week and had enlarged again to 10–15 mm by the 21st day after injection, when biopsy was performed. One of the volunteer recipients of the intradermal lepromin declined to have the nodule removed. It slowly regressed over a two-month period and he remains well, seven years later.

The acid-fast bacilli in the lepromin tests were all found in dense masses of chronic inflammatory cells, including large lymphocytes and giant cells. Occasionally many organisms were present within a single cell, although usually no more than two or three bacilli were present per cell. The dermal nerves and blood vessels in the biopsy site in the normal volunteers were free of organisms.

The normal individuals had been exposed to leprosy patients for periods of more than three months, but all three were in apparent good health. A tuberculin skin test on one of them was positive; the other two tests were negative, although one of these individuals had received BCG ten years previously. None of the volunteers has developed leprosy in the seven years since the tests were performed, and the volunteers who had negative tuberculin skin tests still show negative reactions.

Biopsies of lepromin tests were performed upon patient 1 (Study Period I), patient 3 (Study Periods I and II), and patient 4 (Study Period II). Responses to all of these tests were clinically "negative," although the second test on Patient 3 showed a 3 mm nodule. Of the four lepromin tests biopsied in these three patients, only the second specimen from patient 3 showed a granulomatous response with giant cell formation. In each of the other specimens the injection site contained only a mass of necrotic material in which acid-fast bacilli and lymphocytes, but no giant cells, were observed.

Leprosy bacilli were observed in cutaneous nerves and blood vessels adjacent to the injection site in all three of the leprosy patients tested. These findings contrasted with the firm inflammatory masses containing giant cells observed in the normal "positive" lepromin tests. The organisms in the injected lepromin could be distinguished from endogenous bacilli by their uniform staining quality and pale red aspect. Endogenous bacilli, on the other hand, usually were characterized by bipolar hyperchromicity. In each of the patients tested, bacilli in nerves and blood vessels appeared to be endogenous.

Summary.

The most remarkable discovery made in the evaluation of the skin in the five patients was the finding that no correlation could be made between the clinical appearance of leonine features and the presence of leprosy bacilli. In two patients, enlarged earlobes and classic facies were found to be caused by inflammation around leprosy bacilli. In a third patient, however, bacilli were virtually nonexistent at the moment he suddenly developed similar facies.

This is of great interest: it means that the stage of disease cannot be evaluated on clinical grounds alone, but must be subjected to histologic study. In other words, we cannot assume that all patients with deformed features have equally severe skin involvement with leprosy bacilli.

II. NERVOUS SYSTEM

Physical Examination and Special Functional Tests (Table 3)

The late Dr. James Doull once said that he had never seen a patient with leprosy who did not have some area of disturbed cutaneous sensation. The general rule expressed by Dr. Doull was found to be applicable to the five patients in this study; each one revealed areas of anesthesia and hypesthesia.

Anesthesia or dysesthesia was found to be most extensive in the extremities, where circumferential abnormalities were common. In mapping out the abnormalities, the various observers rarely described identical patterns of sensory loss. The differences were apparently due to several factors:

(1) Apparent variations. This factor is related to fatigue of the patient and the physician, to language barriers, to differences in testing instruments used, and to pressure variations in using the test instruments.

(2) True variations. Disturbance in sensation is related to the stage of disease, which varies with time.

(3) Variation in the loss of individual modalities such as pain, temperature, and touch — which occasionally confused both patient and physician.

Heat and cold perception, two-point discrimination, light touch, pin prick, blunt pressure and deep pain perception were tested in each patient, and no constant pattern of loss or preservation of sensation was observed. In general, light touch and temperature perception were shown to be most extensively affected by the disease while deep pain and pressure perception were generally preserved, but exceptions to these rules were common, especially in the case of patient 2.

Percentage of Body Surface with Abnormal Sensation.

The sensory abnormalities often gave the appearance of a "stocking and glove" distribution. However, it became apparent on close study that the neuropathy showed an irregular border, suggesting localized nerve damage in certain cases, and in other instances following the distribution of major sensory nerves. Characteristic patterns of musculocutaneous and circumflex sensory nerve loss were present in patient 2. Nevertheless, motor loss did not parallel the sensory loss in these mixed nerves.

Recording the extent of anesthesia and hypesthesia on a regular basis was a useful means of assessing the status of the neurologic lesions in these patients. The body surface was evaluated using the "rule of 9's" which is commonly used in calculating the extent of surface injury in burned patients. In this system, 9 percent of the body surface is estimated to be present on the head, 9 percent on each arm, 18 percent on the chest, abdomen and each leg — totalling 99 percent — and 1 percent estimated on the external genitalia.

All patients had measurable sensory defects ranging from 1 percent of the body surface in patient 1 to 64 percent in patient 5 (Figs. 13, 29 and 51). The greatest change observed was that of patient 3, whose sensory deficit *increased* during therapy from 14 percent to 50 percent. As this patient's sensory deficit increased, his bacterial counts actually improved.

Skeletal Muscular Strength.

Monthly observations of the functional capacity of the individual muscles became a valuable record of the progress or regression in the clinical status. Each of 90 muscles or muscle groups was evaluated on a qualitative basis, from normal to zero function. A quantitative estimate was then obtained by scoring "normal" as 5, "good" as 4, "fair" as 3, "poor" as 2, "trace" as 1, and "zero" as 0. Skeletal muscular strength (Table 3) is the ratio of the sums of observed strength and normal strength. For example, if 90 muscle groups were evaluated, the normal strength would be $90 \times 5 = 450$. If five muscles were totally functionless, the observed strength of all muscles would total only $85 \times 5 = 425$. The skeletal muscular strength would then be:

$$425/450 \times 100 = 94.4\%$$

The improvement in patient 2 was documented month after month in records of the therapists' examinations, and the worsening in patient 3 was equally well documented in these examinations. Patient 2 demonstrated a gain in strength from 85 percent to 91 percent during his hospitalization, whereas the loss in patient 3 was from 100 percent to 72 percent. The muscular strength of the five patients ranged from 100 percent in patients, 3, 4 and 5 to lows of 72 to 85 percent in patients 3 and 2.

Electromyogram and Nerve Conduction Time.

Two patients had abnormal electromyograms (EMG). This test provided a means of quantitating the functional deficit more precisely than could be done by tests of muscular strength. The limitations of this technique were evident in its failure to demonstrate an abnormality in patient 1. The reason for failure was apparent: the EMG was performed upon the left ulnar nerve distribution, which was clinically normal, rather than upon muscles innervated by the right ulnar nerve, where weakness and anesthesia were clinically apparent. The EMG test was a painful and frightening experience to the patients, and consequently was not used extensively in the present study. By contrast, the patients enjoyed the therapists' examinations of their muscular strength and it was possible to integrate corrective physical therapy into the testing.

Nerve conduction time (NCT), although a somewhat less painful and frightening test than the EMG, was nevertheless not especially productive of useful information in these patients. The failure of the NCT test was probably due to the psychological inability of the patients to tolerate its repeated use. Prolongation of NCT was detected in two of the patients, as indicated in Table 3.

Peripheral Nerve Lesions.

Enlargement and tenderness of peripheral nerves were observed in four of the five patients (1, 2, 4 and 5). The ulnar, lateral peroneal, posterior auricular, sural and median nerves showed the greatest degree of enlargement on physical examination. In addition, at the time of testicular biopsy it was discovered that patient 2 had a greatly enlarged right external spermatic nerve (approximately 5 mm in diameter). Biopsy of this nerve, which innervates the cremaster muscle and scrotum, revealed considerable chronic inflammation and giant cell formation, although no organisms were found in the nerve. (This patient had relatively few organisms in any of his biopsies.) The other four patients, on the other hand, showed a high density of leprosy bacilli in their cutaneous nerves. No fluctuance was ever palpated in a nerve in these patients, nor was any nerve found to be enlarged to more than three or four times its normal size.

None of the patients developed acute pain or tenderness in nerves during hospitalization. Even patient 3 did not develop painful neuritis, in spite of progressive neuropathy; nerve injections with steroids or hyaluronidase were therefore not performed. No patient showed entrapment syndromes which might have been improved with neurosurgical procedures such as relocation or neurolysis.

All five patients showed abnormalities in the orbital or periorbital nerves or muscles. Patient 1 revealed decreased corneal sensation. Severe lagophthalmos in patient 2 prevented him from closing one of his eyes at night — a peripheral 7th cranial nerve paresis affected the closing of the lower eyelid. Patient 3 developed a moderate degree of lagophthalmos after a four-month profound inflammatory reaction accompanied by fever and peripheral neuritis. Patient 4 demonstrated "possible nodularities" of the corneal nerves; a similar possibility arose in the slit-lamp examination of patient 5, who suffered from a moderate degree of exotropia that interfered with reading or watching television.

Autonomic Nervous System.

Only rarely in leprosy has the autonomic nervous system been found to be diseased, or has the spinal cord been found to contain lepromas or leprosy bacilli such as described in Mitsuda's *Atlas* (1952). One or two exceptions to this generality were noted in this study. The observation that patient 1 voided only once or twice a day led to the performance of two cystometrograms; on both occasions definite abnormalities were found. The patient's bladder accepted 400 ml of warm saline with no effective spontaneous contractions nor was he aware of any uncomfortable sensation. This finding, confirmed by a second cystometrogram, strongly suggests an abnormality in bladder innervation — at least with respect to afferant impulses.

Localized autonomic dysfunction was suggested by the capillary hemorrhages (described above) in patient 2, and by the inability of patients 2 and 5 to produce a seminal emission. In three patients, areas of anhydrosis were observed. No significant abnormalities were detected, however, in cardiac rate or rhythm, gastric or intestinal function, or blood pressure, in any of the five patients.

The neurologic findings in these five patients complement the information obtained on examination of the skin. The patterns of neurologic deficit are similar to those in previous reports, such as those of the World Health Organizaton. These patients illustrate once again the devastation of the nervous system which can occur in leprosy. The remarkable feature of these case studies is the demonstration of extensive functional abnormalities in the early phase of the disease.

III. BACTERIOLOGY AND PATHOLOGY

Distribution and Density of Leprosy Bacilli in Diverse Tissues (Table 4)

Specimens of various kinds were obtained from every easily accessible site, and from several deeper areas of the body, in each patient. These tests were carried out with the full consent and cooperation of the patients and their families. Extensive pathological studies such as these had been reported from necropsies, but to our knowledge had never been performed in living patients with leprosy. Nor had any complete pathologic examinations yet been reported in young patients with indeterminate and dimorphous leprosy.

The present report is, therefore, unique in several respects – the wide variety of tissues examined, the youth of the patients (ages 14 to 26), the early stage of the disease, the sequential observations during a period of natural evolution of the disease, and the grouping of several patients in a single study.

Techniques and Complications.

In each case, biopsies of kidney, latissimus dorsi muscle, Gerota's (perinephric) fat, prostate, testicles, lymph node and skin were obtained while the patient was under general, endotracheal anesthesia. The renal specimens were small wedge biopsies obtained through right flank incisions (percutaneous needle biopsies proved to be inadequate in size and quality for these studies). The testicles were exposed through scrotal incisions; after examination and photographing, seminal vesiculograms and testicular biopsies were obtained. The seminal vesiculograms were obtained with 50% Hypaque® (sodium diazotrite, USP) injected into each vas deferens through #21 needles. Two x-rays of the pelvis were then taken, one immediately, the other five minutes later. The testicular biopsies were small (4 × 1 × 2 mm) wedge biopsies of the surface of the testicles. The testicular and renal incisions were sutured with chromic catgut; Penrose drains were left in the incisions for two days postoperatively. The prostate was biopsied with a Vim-Silverman-Franklin needle introduced in the perineum. The lymph nodes were biopsied by excisions of palpable inguinal nodes.

No major complications were encountered in this surgery. Minor complications included: 1) Delayed wound healing in the flank and scrotal incisions of patient 1, but without wound dehiscence – apparently the result of the development of Lucio arteritis and necrosis of the wound edges. 2) Hematuria following prostatic biopsy (patients 2 and 5). 3) Delayed healing of incisions, and a urinary tract infection, in patient 5. The infection was successfully treated with Gantrisin® (sulfisoxozole).

Lymph node biopsy incisions in patient 5 failed to heal promptly on two separate occasions. Large matted lymph nodes were present in both groins, and a single node was dissected free in each area with difficulty. The incisions became erythematous, with lymphangitis extending for six inches along the saphenous vein. The inflammation responded to warm moist compresses and no antibiotics were used.

Skin biopsies were obtained by surgical excision of tissue using elliptical incisions, or with a 3 mm punch biopsy instrument. Excisional biopsies were divided longitudinally. One fragment was evaluated histologically with hematoxylin and eosin, and Fite stains; the other was emulsified and a smear placed on a glass slide covering approximately 1 cm × 2.5 cm, and stained with Ziehl-Nielssen stain. Tissue sections were evaluated for relative numbers of bacilli on a 0 to ++++ grading system.

Biopsy of the liver was obtained with the Menghini needle in the first biopsy of patient 3 and with the Vim-Silverman-Franklin needle in all other cases, under local anesthesia. In the case of patient 1, hypotension, with a systolic blood pressure of 80–100 for a duration of six hours, was observed following the liver biopsy. (This led to a thorough study of the patient's adrenal function, and because of the finding of diminished responsiveness to ACTH he was treated prophylactically with corticosteroids at the time of his open renal biopsy. He subsequently had no recurrence of hypotension.)

The hypotension in patient 1, and abdominal pain experienced for 24 hours by patient 3, were the only minor complications associated with the six liver biopsies.

Jejunal biopsies were obtained from each patient using the

Crosby capsule. The technique utilized a biopsy instrument on the end of a tube which was swallowed per os and the tip of the tube guided to the proper location under fluoroscopic manipulation. Two specimens were obtained from each patient (one for histology, the other for bacteriologic study). A second pair of specimens was also obtained from patient 5, to confirm the diagnosis of plasmacytosis made on the first specimen. Prothrombin, bleeding and clotting time measurements were made in each patient before biopsy, and after biopsy the patients' hematocrits and feces were examined sequentially for three days. Only one patient (patient 1, Fig. 10) demonstrated any post-biopsy complications, namely melena and a fall in hematocrit from 37 to 32, which subsided spontaneously.

Results.

Histologic examinations of 125 tissue specimens, and bacteriologic examinations of 452 specimens, were performed in this study. Acid-fast bacilli were found in the skin and bone marrow of all five patients. Nasal mucosa, lymph nodes, and liver contained leprosy bacilli in four patients. Testicles and gastric aspirates were next in order of frequency – organisms were present in three patients. Bacilli were found in sputum, spermatic fascia, renal biopsy and seminal or prostatic fluid in two patients.

The patient with diffuse lepromatous leprosy (1) revealed bacilli in his peripheral blood, in the jejunal biopsy, in his deep subcutaneous fat, Gerota's fat, prostate, drainage from the skin ulcerations, buccal mucosa, and hydrocele fluid. Breast tissue and nipple discharge contained leprosy bacilli in patient 4.

It was found that neither the histologic evaluation nor the tissue emulsion was completely satisfactory in detecting small numbers of organisms: occasionally no organisms were seen in one preparation, but were observed in the alternate preparation. A ++++ reading, on the other hand, when present in paraffin sections, was generally seen in tissue emulsions as well. In specimens with low bacterial density, the tissue emulsion was generally more satisfactory than paraffin sections for detection of organisms. Notable exceptions were the renal and prostate biopsies, in which three specimens failed to show organisms in the emulsion but revealed bacilli on a Fite stain of paraffin-embedded sections. On the other hand, the organisms in the first liver biopsy of patient 3 were overlooked in the tissue section but were detected in the emulsion.

Acid-fast bacilli appeared to be associated with significant inflammation, fibrosis or necrosis in the specimens obtained from the nasal mucosa, skin, lymph nodes, subcutaneous fat, spermatic fascia, testicles, and drainage from the ulcerations. The liver biopsy specimens from four patients (1, 3, 4 and 5) contained leprosy bacilli. In three of these patients the bacilli were associated with extensive inflammation and necrosis. However, one of the patients (3) had no inflammatory reaction at the time of the first liver biopsy, and only a slight portal inflammation in the second biopsy.

Bacteria other than *M. leprae* were recovered on eight occasions during the studies. S. *aureus* and ß-hemolytic *streptococcus* were the most common nonspecific organisms detected. This nonspecific bacteriology is tabulated in Table 15. In addition, *M. tuberculosis* was recovered from sputa of patient 5 one year after the studies presented in this monograph were completed. All cultures for tuberculosis had been negative prior to institution of anti-leprosy chemotherapy. The occurrence of pyogenic and tubercular pathogens illustrates the need for vigilance in bacteriologic surveillance of leprosy patients, for serious disability or death may result from super-infections with other microorganisms, if unrecognized and untreated.

Appearance of the Organisms.

Some variation in the density and staining characteristics of the bacilli in separate areas of the body was noted, as mentioned in the discussion of abnormalities of the skin. However, the organisms did not show consistent changes following anti-leprosy chemotherapy, nor did the staining characteristics of organisms in the deep tissues differ significantly from those in the superficial tissues.

Following a discussion with Dr. R. J. W. Rees, we carefully reviewed the specimens from the five patients. There seemed to be more variation of bacilli characteristics between patients, even prior to therapy, than in any one patient at successive stages of his illness or between the various tissues of a patient's body. For example, organisms from patients 1 and 4 always appeared brightly stained and bipolar, regardless of the tissue in which they were located. Faint staining qualities and loss of bipolar hyperchromatic staining was observed in all bacilli in patient 5, whether from skin, lymph nodes, liver or testicles. Faintness of staining was even more pronounced in patient 2. In patient 3 a definite trend toward a loss of acid-fast staining quality was noted during therapy. In no case, however, was a definite distinction apparent between the bacilli in superficial (cool) locations and those in deep (warm) locations, as in the reticuloendothelial system. In all patients the leprosy bacilli in lymph nodes and liver appeared to be as intact and viable as those recovered from skin and testicles.

Comments on Bacilli Found in Venous Blood.

The blood smears were prepared by inserting a needle into a vein and drawing up a few ml of blood into a syringe. A new syringe was then placed on this needle and a few more ml of blood were withdrawn. The needle was then withdrawn from the vein and discarded. Drops of blood were then expressed from the second syringe through a new needle onto each of several slides — as many as six slides in some cases. The slides were numbered in the order in which they were prepared. The blood drops were defibrinated by stirring, as in preparing a "thick film" of blood for examination for malaria parasites. After dehemoglobinization in tap water for twenty minutes, the slides were dried, heat-fixed, and stained by the Ziehl-Niellsen method.

The organisms in the peripheral blood smears of patient 1 were present in clusters (globi) or as isolated organisms. These clusters were often found within large mononuclear cells, apparently monocytes, or were seen in the absence of nuclear material. In the latter instances, the staining qualities of the area around the organisms appeared to be identical to those of leukocytes which lacked nuclei.

In the blood smears obtained prior to therapy in patient 1 as many as seven globi were found in 150 fields examined at 430X. Nine of the thirteen slides prepared from blood of patient 1 contained leprosy bacilli, and all of these nine slides revealed globi — clusters of leprosy bacilli. The density of organisms on the slides was random, and no increased numbers of bacilli were found in the first drops of blood expressed from the syringe compared with the last drops.

The absence of organisms in the peripheral blood of patient 1 after he had received DDS for three months correlates with a report given to us by Dr. John Hanks, who studied the occurrence of leprosy bacilli prior to therapy in patients at Culion Island, Philippine Islands. He compared these patients with similar studies of patients under therapy at the USPHS Hospital at Carville. Although Dr. Hanks' technique of preparing the blood smears was different from that used in the present study, his conclusion was similar: that a decreased number of organisms was seen in the blood of patients who had been treated.

In the present study a similar effort was made to demonstrate bacilli in patient 1 after treatment by examining stained films of the buffy coat of heparinized blood. However, no bacilli were found in these preparations. The disappearance of organisms from the blood after DDS therapy correlated with the disappearance of the organisms from sputum, semen, and gastric washings in patient 1 after three months of DDS therapy.

Renal and Testicular Pathology.

In both patients who had organisms in their renal biopsy specimens, the leprosy bacilli in the kidney were located in the endothelial lining cells of the glomeruli. Reports previous to this study of renal biopsies in patients with leprosy have not revealed organisms, although reports of bacilli in the kidney at necropsy are not uncommon. The present series failed to demonstrate organisms in the tubules, a location reported only by Mitsuda (1952) in necropsies. Apparently an extra-glomerular occurrence of leprosy bacilli in the kidney is unusual.

The testicular specimens which contained leprosy bacilli showed extensive pathologic changes. Patient 1 showed complete destruction of spermatogenesis. The normal tubular and interstitial cells were replaced by macrophages and Virchow cells laden with acid-fast bacilli. In patients 4 and 5, spermatogenesis was present, but bacilli were lying free within the tubules, in the interstitial tissues, and within inflammatory cells in these areas. Spermatogenesis was decreased in these two patients, and fibrosis and atrophy were present, associated with inflammation and infection.

Leydig's interstitial cells were absent in patient 1, and decreased in patients 2, 4 and 5. The Leydig cells are believed to secrete testosterone; thus the reduction in density of these cells may have contributed to the observed decreased 17KS output. This subject is reviewed in Part XII of the Discussion.

Nonspecific Histopathology.

The bacilli in the remainder of the specimens did not appear to be associated with significant pathology, although in some of the specimens additional abnormalities were present. In the jejunal biopsy specimens from patient 5, for example, plasmacytosis was observed. The organisms in the jejunal biopsy of patient 1, however, lay scattered in the cells surrounding the crypts, and did not appear to be associated with plasma cells.

The buccal mucosa of patient 1 contained small collections of organisms in interstitial tissue. Bacteriologic penetration of the oral mucosa and small bowel may be the antecedents to lepromas of the gastrointestinal tract, which have been described at autopsy by Mitsuda. The bacilli in the prostatic specimen of patient 1 were located in the stroma, not associated with inflammation.

A variety of abnormalities were present in bone marrow specimens, such as decreased stainable iron, myeloid hyperplasia, and plasmacytosis. The organisms in the marrow were occasionally in globi, or in smaller collections in macrophages, or appeared as isolated bacilli. Hypertrophy of the breast tissue was present in the specimen obtained from patient 4, but no significant inflammation was associated with the leprosy bacilli in this tissue.

In patient 2, acid-fast bacilli were seen only in the skin and bone marrow. However, granuloma formation, with giant cells of the Langhans type, was prominent in the liver, lymph node, external spermatic nerve, and skin biopsies. Patient 2 had distinctly abnormal testicles, which were large and firm. Testicular biopsy in this case revealed prominent fibrosis and atrophy, and decreased spermatogenesis, although no bacilli could be demonstrated.

Each of the 125 specimens obtained from the five patients was examined for amyloid, using crystal violet stain. No amyloid was found in any specimen, and the only positive staining observed was normal metachromasia which was present in corpora amylacea of the prostate in patient 5.

An Ascaris *Worm with Unusual Features.*

A female specimen of *Ascaris lumbricoides* recovered from patient 5 was studied for acid-fast organisms. The finding of multiple acid-fast, rod-like structures of bacterial size within the ovaries of the cross-sectioned *ascaris* is of uncertain significance. It should be noted, however, that no similar acid-fast material was present in a female *A. lumbricoides* specimen obtained from a 4-year-old negro boy from South Carolina who did not have leprosy. The *ascaris* worm containing acid-fast structures, together with the acid-fast bacilli in the jejunem of patient 1, suggests that leprosy bacilli may pass from the upper to the lower GI tract without structural degradation. Yet, fifteen examinations of the feces in four leprosy patients revealed acid-fast bacilli on only one occasion, in patient 2. Since the density of organisms in this patient was so small, however, it seems unlikely that the organisms in that case were *M. leprae*. It is therefore assumed unlikely that *M. leprae* is excreted in significant numbers in human feces.

Summary.

The widespread distribution of leprosy bacilli in these young men was the most remarkable observation of the entire study. In one case, organisms were recovered in large numbers from many organs of the body and smaller numbers from other areas. In that patient, only skeletal muscle and a scar of the skin were free of organisms. This report further presents the first known cases of leprosy bacilli demonstrated in the kidney and prostate gland prior to death. Considering the youth and healthy appearance of the patients, the extensive destruction and bacillary invasion of skin, lymph nodes, bone marrow, testicles and liver was surprising and impressive.

IV. SKIN TESTS

Dermal Reactivity to Skin Test Antigens in Patients with Leprosy (Table 5)

Previous reports of skin tests in leprosy patients provide conflicting results. Doull (1959) and Guinto (1962) found that more than 50 percent of children in a leprosy endemic area (Cebu, Philippine Islands) who were negative to human and avian tuberculin were positive to lepromin, even in the absence of clinical infection with leprosy. They also reported (1957) that an increase in frequency of positive lepromin reactions after vaccination with BCG could not be attributed to vaccination alone; "natural causes" contributed to the increase. However, analysis of reactions to PPD showed that infection with tuberculosis did not account for the increase in lepromin reactivity.

Jamison and Vollum (1968) reported that positive responses to tuberculin among children of leprous parents were fewer (20 percent) than among children of normal parents (37 percent). They also found that children of leprous parents showed a poor conversion rate after immunization with vole-bacillus vaccine — 17.7 percent as compared to 89.3 percent in children with no family history of leprosy. They suggest that children of leprous parents may have an increased susceptibility to mycobacterial infection.

Guinto and Mabalay (1962) demonstrated a lowering of frequency of tuberculin reactivity in patients with lepromatous leprosy at Cebu, although many necropsy studies — Rogers (1960), Kean (1942), Powell (1955) — have shown a high prevalence of tuberculosis as the cause of death in leprosy. Tuberculosis is reported as the cause of death in 14 to 23 percent of leprosy patients. On the other hand, when Lewis, Fite and Bogen (1961) studied tuberculin reactivity at Carville, they found a high sensitivity to human tuberculin preparations. They did not find an increased frequency of weak positive reactions. However, the patients in the

Carville study were not described in sufficient detail to allow a comparison with the Cebu study.

Recent studies have documented the existence of depressed cellular immune responses in patients with lepromatous leprosy, except in those with erythema nodosum. Bullock (1968) and Waldorf (1966) reported impaired responses to picryl chloride and dinitrochlorobenzene. Turk (1968) demonstrated replacement of the thymus-dependent paracortical areas of lymph nodes in lepromatous leprosy by bacilli-filled, pale-staining reticulo-histiocytes. In spite of these interesting results, no prospective studies have yet been performed which offer a definite answer to the question: Does the depression in cellular responsiveness precede or follow the development of lepromatous leprosy?

Cellular hypersensitivity was studied in the five young leprosy patients by skin tests with eight different antigens. Reactivity was assessed using lepromin, tuberculin, Candidan, Trychophyton, histoplasmin, blastomycin, coccidiodin and Kveim antigens. In general, reactivity was measured before and during therapy in each of the patients except patients 4 and 5, who were studied only prior to therapy. The results of the 55 tests which were performed are shown in Table 5.

Lepromin Test: Medina, Fernandez and Mitsuda Reactions.

The lepromin skin test is generally considered to be a useful procedure in clinical leprology, and the performance of this test upon each patient with leprosy is recommended by most leprologists. The lepromin test is not a diagnostic test for leprosy, but is a means of classifying the responsiveness of a person to the complex mixture of antigens which is termed lepromin. This antigenic mixture was originally described by Mitsuda (1919). Although the techniques used vary somewhat among laboratories, the mixture is essentially a sterile emulsion of lepromas — that is, nodules excised from patients with lepromatous leprosy.

The "lepromina integral" used in our study was provided by the Centro Dermatologico Pascua. It had been prepared in 1959, three years prior to its use in these patients. It was a white, slightly turbid suspension sterilized by tyndallization, and was unchanged in appearance from month to month when stored at either 4° or 20°C.

A positive response to lepromin is a nodule 5 mm or greater, present 21 days after the intradermal injection of 0.1 ml of lepromin. A positive response is observed in 60 to 90 percent of humans, according to Doull (1954, 1959), even among those who reside in nonendemic areas. Positive responses are virtually a sine qua non of tuberculoid leprosy. However, in dimorphous cases – the "borderline" cases of Wade (1940) – and in indeterminate leprosy, the skin test may be positive or negative. In lepromatous leprosy the test is characteristically negative. Indeed, some definitions of the lepromatous type, such as that of the VI International Congress on Leprosy, Madrid, (1953) specify that the lepromin test is always negative in lepromatous leprosy.

Positive reactions to lepromin, with nodules larger than 5 mm at 21 days, were seen in only one of the five patients (2, during therapy), although positive reactions were observed in all three of the normal volunteers tested.

The lepromin test is sometimes evaluated by histological criteria as well as by the size of the nodule. Histologically, the positive reaction is an intense granulomatous, mononuclear inflammation, with phagocytosis of the injected organisms by mononuclear and giant cells. This histologic appearance may be present in cases where the nodule is less than 5 mm in diameter, as in patient 3 of this study. However, in cases where no nodule is present, a giant cell response is rarely seen at the site of injection.

The lepromin skin test may pass through two early stages in its evolution, as described by Medina (1944) and Fernandez (1940). The Medina reaction is a local necrotic process which occurs within a few hours after lepromin injection in patients who have diffuse leprosy of the Lucio type. This was the reaction observed four hours after injection in patient 1. The absence of the Medina reaction in patient 1 after two months of DDS treatment indicated that this reaction is not always present in patients with the Lucio type of leprosy. Fernandez observed that a nodule 5 mm or greater was present at 24 to 72 hours after injection in the majority of patients who later showed a positive nodule at 21 days.

Nodules 5 mm in size or larger were observed in two patients in the present series, and also in the three normal volunteers. The lack of a perfect correlation between the Mitsuda (21 day) and Fernandez (2 to 3 day) reactions is, however, illustrated by the positive Fernandez reaction in patients 3 and 4, who did not have positive Mitsuda reactions at 21 days.

Tuberculin and Fungal Antigens.

Tuberculin tests were performed with purified protein derivative (PPD), supplied by Parke-Davis Co. Blastomycin and histoplasmin were also obtained from Parke-Davis. In each case, the antigen tablets were freshly dissolved in diluent on the day of use. Coccidiodin was obtained from Cutter Laboratories. Trichophyton and Candidan were obtained from Hollister-Stier Laboratories, Philadelphia, Pa., and the stock suspensions were diluted in sterile isotonic saline immediately prior to use.

Only three of the five patients showed reactivity to PPD. None were reactive to blastomycin, histoplasmin and coccidiodin, except for one positive reaction to histoplasmin. The three patients who reacted to PPD showed negative lepromin tests at the time that their PPD reactions were positive. Later, one patient (2) developed a positive lepromin test, while at the same time his PPD — paradoxically — became negative.

Candidan and Trichophyton proved to be particularly satisfactory as skin test agents for measuring delayed hypersensitivity, since four of the five patients responded positively to one or both of these agents. The tests suggested that a definite abnormality in cellular hypersensitivity may be present in diffuse lepromatous leprosy: the only patient who did not develop a typical delayed hypersensitivity reaction to Candidan and Trichophyton was patient 1. This young man was also the only patient who had negative reactions with every other antigen used in skin tests.

The Kveim Test.

A skin test reaction which is positive at 24 to 72 hours is referred to as a "delayed" hypersensitivity reaction. No word has yet come into common usage to describe the prolonged reactions which occur in three special situations: the 21-day positive lepromin reaction, the 14-day reaction of first-set homograft rejection, and the 6-week reaction to Kveim antigen in patients with sarcoidosis. All three of these tests utilize allogenic cells or subcellular fractions: the homograft phenomenon may therefore be a part of the hypersensitivity to both lepromin and Kveim antigens, as well as to standard preparations of homografted cells and tissues. Kveim tests* were performed in two patients on the basis of the clinical and pathological similarities between sarcoidosis and leprosy which were pointed out by James and Jopling (1961). Both patients (4 and 5) exhibited negative lepromin and Kveim tests.

Since the lepromin and Kveim reactions were negative in these two patients with lepromatous leprosy, it is theoretically possible that rejection of homografted tissues would be also impaired in such patients. If tests of skin homograft rejection time in leprosy patients were made, rejection would probably be delayed beyond the usual time of 14 days. In diffuse lepromatous leprosy of the Lucio type, however, skin grafts may show an accelerated (white graft) type of rejection caused by the lepromatous vasculitis which interferes with all wound healing in these patients.

Summary.

The cellular hypersensitivity responses in patients with lepromatous leprosy are remarkable in their differences from responses of normal individuals in that some reactions – such as the lepromin reaction – may be depressed. Normal responses may be observed when other skin test antigens are used, such as tuberculin and fungal antigens. On the whole, however, skin reactivity in diffuse lepromatous leprosy tends to be non-specific and necrotic, in contrast to the erythematous, nodular response, with mononuclear cells, which occurs in tuberculoid leprosy and in humans who do not have leprosy.

* Kveim antigen was kindly furnished by Dr. Lewis Silzbach, Mt. Sinai Hospital, New York City.

V. SEROLOGICAL TESTS

Serological Abnormalities Detected by Immunological Tests (Table 6)

False positive serological reactions and high titer reactivity in a variety of non-specific immunological tests have been reported in previous studies of patients with leprosy. The majority of patients in previous reports (Muelling, 1960, and Cathcart, 1961) have apparently had long-established, chronic infections with leprosy. Those patients differ from the young men in the present study by their more advanced age and by the long period of therapy which most of them had received.

No single test has been reported which is specifically diagnostic for all types of leprosy, although good correlations with lepromatous leprosy were reported by Morris (1961), using the fluorescent-labelled antibody technique, and by Levine (1951), using a tanned cell hemagglutination technique.

It was the purpose of the present study to determine if positive serological reactions correlated well with other data which were being obtained upon the patients. We wished to learn whether a decrease in false positive reactions and a reduction in the titer of non-specific reactions occurred when the patients were treated with antileprosy drugs. Previous reports indicated that a prompt alteration in non-specific serological tests would not be likely to occur after therapy was initiated.

Methods: Twenty Tests Used.

Twenty serological tests performed on 185 occasions in the five patients are reported in this portion of our monograph. Included in the tests were Venereal Disease Research Laboratory Test (VDRL), Kolmer and Treponema Pallidum Immobilization Test (TPI); also the direct Coombs' test, C-reactive protein determination, anti-streptolysin titer, latex agglutination, and heterophile antibody titer. The so-called "febrile agglutinin" responses to salmonella, proteus, brucella and tularemia organisms were measured. Complement fixation tests with blastomycin, coccidiodin, and histoplasmin were performed. The bentonite DNA flocculation test, isohemagglutinins and cold agglutinins were also measured. Other tests performed were: lupus erythematosus (LE) preparations, toxoplasmin dye titer, fluorescent antinuclear antibody tests, and measurement of cryoglobulins and anti-thyroglobulin antibodies. The results of these tests are summarized in Table 6.

Results: Non-specific Reactions were Common.

The findings of greatest interest were false positive VDRL tests in two patients, both of whom also had false positive Kolmer tests. In one of these patients (1), the VDRL was shown to be a false positive reaction by evidence of a negative TPI test. In the other patient (4), the VDRL was presumed to be a false positive reaction when it became negative after treatment with DDS alone; and the patient had never shown signs or symptoms of a primary syphilis infection.

The patient who showed a persistently positive VDRL was also the patient whose biopsies and skin scrapings revealed the greatest number of leprosy organisms. This patient also had the highest globulin (5.9), gamma globulin (4.5), and total protein (9.0) concentration of any of the five patients, as well as more positive serological reactions than any other patient, including a positive direct Coombs' test, blastomycin C.F. reaction, bentonite DNA, heterophile and latex agglutination tests. In contrast, although patient 4 showed a positive VDRL test, he reacted negatively in the Coombs' test, bentonite DNA, heterophile and latex agglutinations. The VDRL reaction in this patient became negative during DDS therapy.

The three patients (1, 4 and 5) most extensively involved with leprosy bacilli showed positive C-reactive protein determinations. No significant changes occurred in these results during Study Period II, when the patients were receiving anti-leprosy chemotherapy.

Antistreptolysin titers were positive at some point in the hospitalization of each patient. The only patients with titers of 500 units or more were patients 1 and 5 prior to therapy, and patient 3 during his inflammatory reaction (Study Period III). Each patient recorded one or more positive reactions in the "febrile agglutinins," but none showed unusually high titers or significant changes during hospitalization. Highest in any of the five patients was a titer of 1:400 with salmonella E in patient 4. The iso-hemagglutinins were positive in all patients except patient 1, whose blood type was AB, and who would not normally have iso-hemagglutinins (anti-A or anti-B). High titers of iso-hemagglutinins were seen in patients 4 and 5 (both 1:512), and a rising titer was observed in patient 3 during the period of his inflammatory reaction (anti-B increased from 1:32 to 1:256).

The toxoplasmin dye titer was positive at greater than 1:1,000 in patient 2, who had extensive chronic chorioretinitis. This test was performed in two additional patients — one of whom had minimal chorioretinitis — and was negative in both of the remaining two patients. It was concluded that patient 2 probably had had toxoplasmosis in the past, and that this possibly caused his chorioretinitis. It is interesting to speculate that the diffuse granulomatosis demonstrated in biopsies of patient 2 may represent healed or healing infections with any or all of three diseases: toxoplasmosis, tuberculosis and leprosy.

Prognostic Value of the Tests.

It became apparent that nonspecific serological reactions do provide a useful means of assessing both the prognosis and current state of the disease in many patients. That is, a high titer of nonspecific or false positive reactions *usually* represented a state of high bacterial density in the five patients tested. However, patient 3 was a very important exception to this rule: his increasing titer of iso-hemagglutinins in Study Period III was not related to an increase in bacterial density, but was associated instead with a diffuse inflammatory reaction and a *decrease* in bacterial density.

The titer of nonspecific reactions and false positive reactions correlated well with the level of serum proteins, particularly globulin and gamma globulin. The changes in serum proteins and protein fractions are described in the next part of the discussion. It was concluded that accurate determination of total serum protein, and measurement of protein fractions by paper electrophoresis provided a satisfactory quantitation of changes which were reflected qualitatively by nonspecific serological determinations.

VI. SERUM PROTEINS

A Decrease in Total Globulin and Immunoglobulin Concentration was Correlated with Bacteriologic Improvement, but the Reverse was not Necessarily True. (Table 7)

Elevation of the serum globulin concentration has previously been reported to occur in leprosy. Muelling (1960) found that a decrease in serum mucopolysaccharide concentration was apparently correlated with clinical improvement in lepromatous leprosy. The five patients in the present series were studied with serial determinations of the serum proteins and protein fractions to determine if abnormal findings were present in the early stages of leprosy. When abnormalities were detected, efforts were made to determine how they related to the clinical status of the patients.

Methods.

Total protein was determined by the biuret method; albumin was measured by differential precipitation in salt solution, and globulin was calculated as an arithmatic difference. Other serum protein fractions were estimated by paper electrophoresis, by electrophoresis in agar and starch gels, by immunoelectrophoresis, and by an immuno-radioisotopic technique.

Total serum protein concentration in the five patients was measured at one to three week intervals, on a total of 117 occasions. Estimation of gamma globulin concentration by paper electrophoresis was performed on 68 occasions. The values in each study period remained remarkably constant for each patient, although occasional variations were observed which were consistent with laboratory errors. In reporting maximum and minimum levels for each patient the effect of laboratory error has been diminished by a calculation of the mean values for each treatment period. The data presented in this section of the report are, therefore, based on these mean values of total protein, albumin, globulin and gamma globulin. These data are summarized in Table 7.

Results: Elevation in IgG, IgA and IgM Globulins.

The serum protein concentration was found to be greater than normal in only one patient (1), whose mean total protein concentration was 9.1 gm per 100 ml in Study Period I, and 8.7 in Study Period II. A high-normal value was present in one other patient (5), who showed a total protein of 7.8. These two patients, and patient 4, revealed elevated serum globulin levels; the pretreatment mean levels ranged from 3.7 (patient 4) to 5.9 (patient 1). Patients 1 and 4 demonstrated decreased albumin levels, 3.2 and 2.9 respectively. During his inflammatory reaction in Study Period III, patient 3 also developed a low albumin and elevated globulin, with a reversed A/G ratio of 2.9/3.8. A/G ratio in this case is the average of 16 determinations of serum proteins over a period of four months.

The patients with elevated serum globulins were found to have elevation of the gamma globulin, (γ globulin, IgG) as revealed by paper, starch gel and immunoelectrophoretic techniques (Figs. 88, 89, 90). Mean values determined by paper electrophoresis prior to therapy on the three patients with elevated total globulin and gamma globulin ranged from 1.9 (patient 4) to 4.5 (patient 1).

It should be emphasized that a gamma globulin level of 4.5 gm per 100 ml of non-myeloma globulin is a truly remarkable concentration. This value is the mean of four determinations performed over a two-month period. An elevation of gamma globulin also appeared to be present in patient 3, based on immuno-radioisotopic analysis* at the end of Study Period I when the total globulin was still normal, and before an increased gamma globulin was detected on paper electrophoresis.

A sharp, dense IgM line (beta-2-macroglobulin, B2M) was detected on immunoelectrophoresis of the serum of patients 1, 3, 4 and 5, and an elevation of this serum fraction was confirmed by the immuno-radioisotopic titrations which were performed in patients 1 and 3. A sharp, dense IgA line (beta-2-A globulin, B2A) was present in the immunoelectrophoresis of the serum of patients 1, 3 and 4. Immuno-radioisotopic titrations confirmed the elevated level of IgA protein in patients 1 and 3. The immuno-radioisotopic test was not performed on the sera of patients 4 and 5.

* By Dr. John Fahey

The sharp, dense IgM and IgA lines seen in the immunoelectrophoreses of the leprosy patients' sera were definitely greater than normally are present. However, exact quantitation of the amounts of these proteins in sera was not obtainable from immunoelectrophoretic analysis of serum. This test was primarily useful for its qualitative description of abnormalities.

Although serum protein abnormalities were detected in four of the five patients, none of the techniques used were successful in distinguishing any chemical or immunochemical abnormalities in these proteins. The precipitation and electrical mobility of the serum proteins appeared normal, with no suggestion of myeloma or other abnormal types. The "Australia antigen" which Blumberg (1967) first described in 1965 has recently been reported to be associated with lepromatous leprosy in Cebu. This unusual α-lipoprotein was not sought in our studies in 1962–63. The serum protein abnormalities in our five leprosy patients appeared to be quantitative rather than qualitative. This conclusion is not contradicted by the immunoelectrophoretic findings, for the precipitin levels found in those tests were in the positions of migration of normal serum IgA and IgM proteins.

Decrease in Serum Globulins during Therapy.

Serial determinations of the serum proteins did not reveal a consistent pattern in all of the patients of either stability or change. However, it was of interest that patients 1, 2 and 3 showed clinical improvement in Study Period II and exhibited slight, gradual lowering in the serum globulin level. Observed decreases in mean values were 0.4, 0.6 and 0.8 gm per 100 ml respectively. These were decreases of 4.4 percent, 8.5 percent, and 10.5 percent (Table 7 and Figs. 10, 31 and 46).

Study Period II was a time of recurrent erythema nodosum reaction in patient 4, as depicted in Fig. 67. This persistent inflammation was presumably the reason that this patient did not have a decrease in his serum globulin level during therapy, but on the contrary exhibited a small increase, from 3.7 to 3.9.

In patients 1 and 3 the changes in gamma globulin levels during Study Period II from 4.5 to 3.6, and from 1.5 to 0.9, respectively, represented decreases of 20 percent and 40 percent. In patients 2 and 4 no significant change in gamma globulin concentration was detected during Study Period II. However, inspection of the clinical chart (Fig. 31) of patient 2 shows that gamma globulin had gradually decreased to its lowest level at the conclusion of Study Period II, after five months of DDS therapy.

During the inflammatory reaction of patient 3 (Study Period III), the serum albumin became abnormally low, and the serum total globulin and gamma globulin levels became greater than normal. The decrease in serum albumin was believed to be due to decreased synthesis and increased catabolism or gastrointestinal loss of albumin rather than to urinary loss: although proteinuria was present, the urinary loss averaged 0.5 gm per day, and never exceeded 0.8 gm per day.

Paper electrophoretic determinations of alpha and beta globulins, and starch gel determination of glyco- and lipo-proteins, failed to reveal any consistent abnormalities in the patients in this series.

Recapitulation.

In summary, the abnormalities of the serum proteins in the five leprosy patients in the present report were:

1) Elevation of the immunoglobulins – IgG, IgA and IgM and and total gamma globulin.
2) Decreased serum albumin in two patients.
3) Normal or elevated levels of total serum protein.
4) A gradual decrease in serum globulin and gamma globulin during therapy in the patients who showed general clinical stability or improvement.

The patient whose serum proteins were most abnormal was the patient who had shown the most extensive penetration with leprosy bacilli. In another patient, a three-month period of apparent clinical improvement was accompanied by a slight decrease in serum globulin and gamma globulin levels. This period was followed by a febrile reaction in which bacteriologic improvement occurred but the total globulin and gamma globulin levels increased once again. The patient with the fewest leprosy bacilli present showed no consistent abnormality in his proteins.

In spite of the interesting correlations which existed between clinical status and serum proteins, it must be concluded that studies of the serum proteins did not contribute as much to the management and understanding of the patients' illnesses as was learned from bacteriologic studies and physical examination.

VII. OPHTHALMOLOGY

Diseases of the Eye Associated with Leprosy (Table 8)

Blindness has long been regarded as one of the most dreaded complications of leprosy, vividly portrayed in the legend of Troilus and Cressida.* In the sentence passed by the gods upon the wanton Cressida:

"From health of body I thee now deprive,
And to thy sickness there shall be no cure,
But in dolour thy days to endure.

Thy crystal eyes mingled with blood I make,
Thy voice so clear, unpleasant, weak and hoarse;
Thy lusty complexion o'erspread with spots black,
And vivid lumps appearing in thy face.
Where thou comest, each man shall flee the place;
Thus shalt thou go begging from house to house,
With cup and clapper, like one lazarous."

Much later, as her life draws to a close, the blind Cressida is unable to recognize Troilus, and when her former lover passes by,

". . . upon him she cast up both her eyes.
And with a glance it came into his thought
That he sometime her face before had seen;
But she was in such plight he knew her nought."

Prevention and therapy of ocular complications are major challenges in the treatment of leprosy. A complete ophthalmologic evaluation was not only a necessary part of the present research project, but was of great importance to the individual patients. It was of interest, of course, to be able to compare the ophthalmologic findings with the findings in each of the many other organs and systems which were studied.

The techniques used in this study were the standard procedures of ophthalmologic examination, with particular attention to the corneal nerves as viewed by slit-lamp examination. After careful physical examination the conjunctivae were scraped gently

* Larkey, S. V. 1961.

and the scrapings examined for acid-fast bacilli. The examinations were performed soon after admission of the patients to the hospital and were repeated no later in each case than six months thereafter. Whenever symptoms developed during hospitalization, interim examinations were performed. In the case of each patient, on physical or laboratory examination major abnormalities were apparent.

Serious Ophthalmological Problems in All Five Patients.

Patient 1 was greatly disturbed by the almost total alopecia of his eyebrows and eyelashes. Physical examination of this patient also revealed a decrease in sensation of the cornea, and thickened conjunctivae.

Patient 2 had severe lagophthalmos of the right eye due to a peripheral facial nerve palsy, resulting in inability to close the eyelids completely. At the time he was admitted to the hospital he suffered from severe conjunctivitis. His right eye was painful, and his vision had decreased to 20/200. The slit-lamp examination of that eye revealed no corneal abrasions or thickened nerves; the symptoms responded promptly to methyl cellulose eye drops, given several times daily. Cause of the decreased visual acuity in this patient was never determined with certainty. He was found to have extensive chorioretinitis, however, which appeared inactive on funduscopic examination. These lesions were more extensive in the right eye than in the left.

This patient had experienced visual problems in his right eye for several years, which he said worsened after the eyelids failed to close completely. On the basis of the lack of previous reports of choroid or retinal involvement with leprosy, it is assumed unlikely that this patient had leprous chorioretinitis. He did show a toxoplasmin dye titer of > 1:1000, and his retinal lesions were entirely consistent with toxoplasmosis. In summary, patient 2 exhibited decreased visual acuity due to chronic chorioretinitis, probably from toxoplasmosis. His vision was further compromised by conjunctivitis due to inability to close the eyelids as a result of leprous neuritis of the seventh cranial nerve.

Patient 3, whose only abnormality on initial physical examination was a small area of healed chorioretinitis, developed conjunctivitis and a mild left lagophthalmos on two occasions during the reaction which occurred in Study Period III. On both occasions the conjunctivitis subsided promptly during systemic prednisone therapy. The lagophthalmos was minimal, being apparent only on careful physical examination and never symptomatic to the patient.

Patient 4 had a recurrent area of erythema nodosum in the lateral portion of the left eyebrow. Swelling and pain in this nearly hairless area accompanied each of his monthly febrile episodes. On several occasions his eyelid was closed almost completely by adjacent edema of the eyebrow. On another occasion, he developed a small sty on the inner aspect of the lid, completely hidden from external examination, coincident with an erythema nodosum lesion immediately adjacent to the eyelid. When the sty was finally discovered it responded promptly to warm soaks, and no progressive damage from the recurrent inflammations could be detected. His vision appeared to be normal, but the corneal nerves were believed "possibly" to be slightly thickened. The ophthalmoscopic examination was otherwise normal.

Patient 5 showed acid-fast bacteria in conjunctival scrapings, although similar examinations in the other four patients were negative. Patient 5 also had "possible" thickening of the corneal nerves. He showed a symptom of major disability probably unrelated to leprosy, namely dysopia due to bilateral exotropia. This prevented him from reading or watching television without developing a headache.

In summary, major ophthalmological abnormalities were detected in all five patients; in each, at least some of these abnormalities were due to leprosy. Additional abnormalities which were probably unrelated to leprosy were: chronic or healed chorioretinitis in two patients, a sty in a third patient, and symptomatic exotropia in another patient. The only treatments given for the patients' ophthalmologic problems were: methyl cellulose for conjunctivitis, and warm soaks for the sty. In addition, one patient was treated with oral corticosteroids for a severe febrile reaction, and concurrently existing conjunctivitis subsided promptly.

Lesions of the eye and its adjacent structures found to be specifically due to leprosy were: alopecia of the eyelashes and eyebrows in two patients, thickening of the corneal nerves or diminished corneal sensation in three, acid-fast bacilli in conjunctival scrapings in one, and lagophthalmos due to inflammation of the facial nerve in two patients.

VIII. HEMATOLOGICAL ABNORMALITIES

Anemia, Leukopenia, Thrombocytopenia, Hypersplenism, Periodic Hemolysis, Poor Iron Absorption and Leprosy of the Bone Marrow were Studied (Table 9)

Abnormalities of peripheral blood, hematopoetic system and reticuloendothelial system have been described and discussed by a number of previous authors, including Cochrane (1959), Derbes (1961), Dogliotto (1960), Black (1938), and Mitsuda (1937, 1952). It has been reported, for example, that leprosy bacilli are found in the reticuloendothelial system in patients with lepromatous leprosy, especially in the spleen, lymph nodes and liver. Abnormalities of the bones and bone marrow have been emphasized by Lechat. Histologic studies have revealed leprosy bacilli in blood vessels in tissue sections, and many authors assume that the disease is most likely disseminated by blood and lymphatic spread. Occasional reports of leprosy bacilli in the peripheral blood are also encountered, although this phenomenon is not generally appreciated.

Anemia is often reported to occur in patients with leprosy, and much mystery surrounds its origin. Sulfones have been implicated by some investigations as a cause of the anemia, since it is known that methemoglobinemia can result from toxic doses of sulfones and a mild hemolytic reaction has been suspected in patients receiving even small doses. Glucose-6-phosphate dehydrogenase deficiency was found by Kher in Nagpur, India, to be more prevalent in patients with leprosy than in normal individuals. He concluded that sulfone toxicity may lead to hemolysis in patients with G-6PD deficiency.

Under field conditions, with outpatient therapy, and even in leprosaria, many causes for anemia are possible: malnutrition, iron deficiency, and other infections – particularly tuberculosis, intestinal parasites and malaria. It is obvious that no single cause can be assumed to be the explanation for anemia in any patient with leprosy; a careful history and physical examination, and complete analysis of all pertinent laboratory examinations must be carried out in order to understand the origins of anemia. The present study demonstrates that if the anemia is of complex origin, or if the degree of anemia and its causes are not constant, even the most complete study may fail to give a clear answer to the problem.

Methods.

Regular estimations of the circulating red cell mass were performed in each patient. Hematocrit tests were performed at least two to three times weekly. Occasionally, longer periods elapsed between determinations, although daily tests were performed when specifically indicated. Hemoglobin and RBC counts were performed at weekly intervals during critical periods. Platelet counts and reticulocyte counts were performed every one to two weeks, and white blood cell counts and differential counts were performed at weekly intervals.

In four of the five patients, daily WBC counts were performed for several days following the open renal biopsy, to measure the leukocyte response to major surgery. Erythrocyte sedimentation rate (ESR) was measured weekly by the Westergren method, and the serum iron was measured every two to three months. For each patient, three to six fecal specimens were examined for occult blood; at least an equal number of examinations were made for intestinal ova and parasites. Bone marrow aspirations were performed before and during therapy on each patient, and additional examinations were performed from time to time. These specimens were stained for study of the blood cells and their precursors, for iron, and for acid-fast bacilli. A tissue block was also prepared for each specimen, sectioned, and stained for acid-fast bacilli.

Blood sulfone determinations were performed upon three of the patients using the Bratton-Marshall method to study the relationship between sulfone level and the peripheral blood counts. Each patient was tested with Cr^{51} studies of blood volume, red cell mass, and red cell half-life. In one case — the only patient with detectable splenomegaly — the splenic uptake of Cr^{51} was measured with a surface Geiger counter, following the intravenous injection of labelled red cells (Fig. 24). Bleeding time and clotting time were measured in all patients; erythrocyte glucose-6-phosphate dehydrogenase was measured in one patient.

Urine and fecal urobilinogen was measured at least once in each patient, at a time when anemia was present; several measurements were usually made of these levels. Urinary excretion of urobilinogen was measured over a two hour period. Fecal urobilinogen was calculated on a 24-hour basis, using three consecutive 24-hour collection periods. Osmotic fragility of the red cells was measured one or more times in each patient, at a time when anemia was present.

In general, mean values in each study period are reported, except in instances where the abnormality was short-lived. In all cases, the sudden development of unusual or unexpected values was confirmed by one or more additional determinations to rule out the possibility of laboratory error. For example, investigation of unexpected alterations in blood counts led to measurement of the hematocrit 83 times in patient 4 and 55 times in patient 1. Other values checked by frequent determinations were, for example, in patient 1: hemoglobin (50 times), RBC count (16 times), platelet count (27 times), reticulocytes (30 times), WBC count (57 times) and erythrocyte sedimentation rate (42 times). Table 9 summarizes the examinations from all five patients.

Results.

All five patients demonstrated significant abnormalities in their peripheral blood studies. All were anemic at some time during the study; all had elevated sedimentation rates. Leukopenia was present in two patients, and persistent thrombocytopenia was observed in one patient. Serum iron was low in three patients, one of whom failed to improve with oral iron therapy. Acid-fast bacilli were present in the bone marrow of each of the five patients at some time during hospitalization.

Anemia.

The degree of anemia ranged from moderate in patient 5 to severe in patient 4. The minimum hematocrit in patient 5 was 37; the minimum hematocrit in patient 4 was 26. The anemia spontaneously disappeared during therapy in patient 4, with a rise in hematocrit to 45, and was most distressing in patient 3, whose hematocrit gradually fell to 33 during the febrile reaction in Study Period III. This anemia failed to respond to oral iron therapy, steroids, or vitamins. In every case the anemia was microcytic and hypochromic.

One of the patients (1) was continuously anemic and showed little improvement while on therapy. His maximum hematocrit was only 39, his minimum hematocrit 32, and his mean value 35. An *increase* in the reticulocyte count of this patient during therapy suggested that the rate of red cell destruction may have increased due to sulfones. Prior to institution of therapy, reticulocytes ranged from 0.2 to 1.2 percent. On DDS therapy reticulocytes increased to a maximum of 5.0 percent.

Patient 3 developed a progressive anemia during his hospitalization. The anemia began during Study Period I, when hematocrit fell from 47 to 37, and increased during sulfone therapy, when hematocrit fell from 43 to 34. The anemia became severe during his febrile reaction and subsequent convalescence: hematocrit fell from 38 to 33. Mean hematocrit in these three study periods fell sequentially from 45 to 38 to 35. Because the anemia was microcytic and hypochromic, it was considered possibly due to blood loss or iron deficiency. Withdrawal of blood from the patient was for this reason restricted to a minimum and he was given oral iron therapy for prolonged periods of time.

When bone marrow and serum in patient 3 failed to show an increase in iron, his anemia was judged to be due partially to failure of iron absorption. Serum iron actually fell from 65 to 29 gamma per 100 ml during the time he received ferrous sulfate by mouth in Study Period III. During the period of greatest anemia he demonstrated a diminished reticulocytosis and a low serum iron. Reticulocytes were only 2.0 percent of the total red cells, and the mean value was only 1.0 percent during Study Period III.

Sedimentation rate in patient 3 (corrected for hematocrit level) increased, as the anemia became more severe, from a maximum of 40 in Study Period I to 55 in Study Period II, and to a peak value of 60 in Study Period III. The high sedimentation rate suggested that erythropoesis may have been impaired by fever and inflammation as well as by decreased iron stores.

The patient showed a decreased red cell mass (24.5 ml per kg) at a time when anemia was present; yet total blood volume appeared normal at this time (70.0 ml per kg), and red cell survival time was normal, with a half-life of 28 days (Fig. 60). At the time of the Cr^{51} study sulfone therapy had been discontinued, and the patient's blood sulfone level had fallen to zero. He showed a normal urobilinogen excretion, normal red cell osmotic fragility, no fecal or urinary blood loss, and a negative Coombs' test.

All data considered, the anemia in patient 3 was apparently due to a failure of erythropoesis resulting from decreased intestinal iron absorption and/or impaired bone marrow function. Other factors may have played a role, such as the earlier therapy with sulfones, the inflammatory reaction associated with leprosy, or the diphenyl thiourea therapy which he received in Study Period III.

Patient 4 revealed a particularly interesting form of anemia which showed a cyclical periodicity and was apparently of compound origin. Early in his hospitalization the regularity of his febrile reactions, accompanied by erythema nodosum, was not fully recognized. As the pattern became clear, however, it was observed that each reaction was associated with weight loss, anemia, fever, leukocytosis, elevation in sedimentation rate, and the development of new erythema nodosum lesions. It was further noted that the reactions occurred at approximately 4 to 5-week intervals and lasted 10 to 14 days. The reactions subsided gradually, more or less spontaneously. They are illustrated in Fig. 67 and Table 16.

During each reaction, patient 4 received supportive therapy in the form of aspirin, sedatives, antibiotics, antihistamines, and chloroquine. Although the supportive therapy varied in type and dosage, the pattern of the reactions showed little variation. The least severe of the reactions developed in February-March immediately following the open renal biopsy. Endogenous production of ACTH due to the stress of surgery may have aborted this reaction.

Studies of Cr^{51} red cell survival and blood volume in patient 4 were performed during two of his reactions (Fig. 71). The Cr^{51} studies were begun at the time of maximum anemia; at that time red cell mass was decreased, blood volume was normal and red cell survival was normal. The patient showed an increased reticulocyte count during the period of recovery from each reaction. Additional studies for hemolysis were negative, including determinations of serum bilirubin, urine urobilinogen and Coombs' tests.

The possibility that anemia in patient 4 was due to water intoxication was ruled out in view of the normal total blood volume at a time when anemia was maximal. If anemia had been caused by hemodilution he would have shown a normal red cell mass and a greater than normal total blood volume. It was further observed that hematocrit declined simultaneously with body weight loss during each reaction. If water intoxication had been the cause of anemia, a decrease in weight — due to loss of water — would have occurred as the hematocrit increased during the recovery phase after each febrile reaction.

White Blood Cells.

Leukopenia was most severe in patient 2, who showed a minimum WBC of 2,500 and a mean WBC of 3,400 in Study Period II. After renal biopsy, however, his WBC showed a normal transient elevation to 8,500. The chronic leukopenia of patient 1, on the other hand, did not change with ACTH, renal biopsy, or gastrointestinal hemorrhage due to jejunal biopsy. The maximum WBC of patient 1 was reported as 6000; but this value was not confirmed and was apparently spurious. His mean WBC was only 3200 in Study Period I and 3000 in Study Period II.

The leukopenia in patient 1 was most likely due to hypersplenism, especially inasmuch as splenic trapping of Cr^{51} was demonstrated following injection of labelled red cells. This patient's enlarged spleen probably contained large numbers of leprosy bacilli, for hyperplasia of the reticuloendothelial system and massive infiltration with acid-fast bacilli were demonstrated in biopsies of his liver and lymph nodes. Hypersplenism could not be demonstrated in patient 2, in spite of the documentation of chronic leukopenia. However, few organisms were detected in smears and biopsies in patient 2 and he did not have gross splenic enlargement.

Patient 2 did have granulomatous disease of the liver and lymph nodes; he had testicular fibrosis, chorioretinitis, a positive tuberculin skin test, and a positive toxoplasmin dye titer. It is possible, then, that he did have a functional form of hypersplenism as a result of chronic toxoplasmosis or tuberculosis but without enlargement of the spleen. Or perhaps a somewhat enlarged spleen was present, but oriented transversely and difficult to detect on physical examination. In summary, no definite etiology for the leukopenia in patient 2 was apparent.

Platelets.

Thrombocytopenia was observed, in addition to anemia and leukopenia, in patient 1. This finding was presumably due to the hypersplenism, or possibly in some degree to the chronic bacteremia with leprosy bacilli observed during Study Period I. In this case the mean platelet count varied only slightly before and after therapy, being 134,000 in Study Period I and 120,000 in Study Period II. In contrast, the mean platelet counts of the other four patients were normal, ranging from 201,000 in patient 2 to 410,000 in patient 4.

Sedimentation Rate.

Erythrocyte sedimentation rate (ESR) was elevated at some time in all five patients. Maximum ESR values were 60, 80, 100, 110, and 122 in the five patients. In each, with the exception of patient 5, the ESR declined appropriately during periods of apparent clinical improvement. The exception was probably due to the shorter period of observation in the case of patient 5 — three months in contrast to six to nine-month periods of observation of the others.

Mean ESR fell during therapy in patient 1 from 97 to 87, in patient 2 from 27 to 3, and in patient 3 from 10 to 8 (before his febrile reaction began). Inflammatory responses in patient 3 (Study Period III) were associated with elevation of mean ESR to 33 and in patient 4 (Study Period II) with an elevation in mean ESR value to 60. ESR thus became a useful laboratory determination in assessing the patients' clinical status.

ESR elevation did not always indicate worsening of the bacteriologic status, but served as a signal to observe the patient for an inflammatory reaction. In patient 1, the ESR was consistently elevated until therapy was begun, then occasional transient decreases began to appear. ESR values as low as 20 were recorded on several occasions during Study Period II in this patient. In patient 2, the ESR was normal during the pre-treatment observation period but declined to extremely low levels during therapy, showing minimum values of 2–3. The ESR in patient 3 was normal before therapy and continued normal during sulfone treatment. After a reaction began, the ESR elevated persistently. The cyclical changes in ESR in patient 4 are discussed elsewhere in this monograph. The ESR in patient 5 was elevated during the entire period of pre-treatment observation. In summary, ESR proved to be a simple, inexpensive means of evaluating clinical status. A decreasing or low ESR was universally associated with bacteriologic improvement and a good clinical response.

Serum Iron.

Values of serum iron as low as 29–39 μgm per 100 ml were observed in three patients, while the other two showed mean serum iron values in the normal range (63–144). Two of the patients (1 and 4) who had initially demonstrated low values showed a rise in serum iron when treated with oral iron preparations, and mean values in these cases rose as high as 90. The poor iron absorption in patient 3 has been discussed.

Normal Results.

The remainder of the hematologic studies as outlined above showed no significant abnormalities. Results are summarized in Table 15. Specifically, no abnormalities were found in differential white blood cell counts, bleeding time, clotting time, urine or fecal urobilinogen excretion, osmotic fragility or red cell glucose-6-phosphate dehydrogenase.

Summary

Anemia in leprosy is once again demonstrated to be a multifaceted problem. The patients in this study exemplified at least three different forms of anemia: hemolysis, impaired marrow function and poor iron absorption. An additional suspect as a contributory cause of anemia was sulfone toxicity. Leukopenia was unexpectedly present in two patients, and all of the patients had leprosy bacilli in their bone marrow. Leprosy bacilli were recovered in peripheral blood specimens in one patient prior to therapy; this chronic bacteremia may have contributed to thrombocytopenia. Hypersplenism, documented by trapping of Cr^{51} labelled red blood cells, was discovered in the patient who demonstrated leprosy bacteremia.

IX. LIVER, STOMACH AND INTESTINES

SEVERE HISTOLOGIC CHANGES WERE FOUND IN THE LIVER. MALNUTRITION WAS PRESENT THOUGH MILD. AMYLOIDOSIS WAS ABSENT (TABLE 10)

The liver and gastrointestinal tract have previously been described as abnormal in many patients with leprosy. The abnormalities have been recognized as due either to specific destruction of tissues by leprosy bacilli and adjacent inflammation, or to lesions associated with leprosy such as tuberculosis, amyloidosis and parasitic diseases.

Introduction.

Postmortem studies by Mitsuda (1952) in patients with leprosy revealed leprous hepatic necrosis, oral and hypopharyngeal ulceration, and lepromas of the stomach. Nonspecific lesions of the gastrointestinal tract found to be associated with leprosy include hyperglobulinemia and malnutrition. Secondary amyloidosis may be severe enough to cause malabsorption, a sprue-like syndrome, hypoproteinemia and death. Renal amyloidosis was the most common cause of death at Carville prior to 1950, according to Beddow and Tilden (1960). Hyperglobulinemia occurs in a wide variety of inflammatory processes, causing nonspecific changes in the so-called "liver function tests" (cephalin flocculation, and thymol turbility). Malnutrition occurs in untreated, advanced cases, and in outcasts who are consciously neglected by their communities. Malnutrition is accentuated by intestinal parasites, tuberculosis, malaria, drug reactions, loss of extremities, and blindness.

History and Physical Examination.

Although significant gastrointestinal abnormalities were previously described in association with advanced leprosy, it was unknown if the early stages of leprosy were associated with abnormal gastrointestinal function. Careful study of the five young men demonstrated only minimal clinical evidence of abnormalities in this system.

The five patients had all lived on diets which were monotonous but nutritious. None had been hungry for more than a day or two at any time, and starvation had never been imminent in any of their families. The diets were predominantly of vegetable origin, the tortilla being the most common item. Two of the patients (3 and 4) were slender and appeared younger than most young men of their ages in the United States. Neither of the two gained more than a few kilograms in weight during hospitalization, and it was concluded that their small stature was possibly due to heredity rather than to leprosy or malnutrition. One of the patients (5) was large-boned, heavy, and somewhat obese, although his diet had been the poorest of all five patients.

None of the patients had ever noticed any abnormalities in digestion, other than occasional transient gastroenteritis, and they said their feces were normal. None had ever been aware of the passage of worms or blood in the stools, and none had bulky foul-smelling stools, abdominal pain or jaundice. All expressed a preference for Mexican cooking, fresh früits and vegetables, and meats cooked with spices and peppers, as opposed to boiled vegetables and meats with cream sauces.

The single patient who revealed a significant abnormality on physical examination of the gastrointestinal system was patient 1, who had hepatosplenomegaly. His liver edge was 6 cm inferior to the right costal margin, and the spleen tip was 12–16 cm inferior to the left costal margin.

Studies Performed.

Laboratory examinations performed to evaluate the liver and gastrointestinal tract included biopsies of liver, gum and jejunem, and examination of the feces for ova, parasites, acid-fast bacilli and blood. Other studies included upper gastrointestinal x-rays, barium enema examinations, and gastric washings for acid-fast bacilli. Serum and plasma specimens were studied for cholesterol (total and free), proteins, thymol turbidity, cephalin flocculation, glutamic oxalacetic transaminase, glutamic pyruvic transaminase, Vitamin A, carotene, triglycerides and phospholipids. In each of these tests, abnormalities were discovered in one or more patients. In prothrombin time, alkaline phosphatase and BSP tests, performed in all patients, an abnormality was discovered in each examination in at least one patient. A refractory low serum iron was discovered in one patient. Studies performed in all patients for amyloidosis, serum lactic dehydrogenase, and bilirubin were normal. Normal oral tolerance to glucose and D-xylose was found in all cases, as well as normal serum calcium and phosphorus values. Transient positive values for occult blood in the feces were found, whereas examinations of stool fat were normal on all occasions.

Microscopic Examination: Pathology and Parasitology.

In spite of the apparent normality of the liver and gastrointestinal tracts on history and physical examinations, significant abnormalities were detected on histologic study. All five patients demonstrated abnormal liver biopsies and intestinal parasites. Four of the liver biopsies showed acid-fast bacilli; hepatic destruction by necrosis and fibrosis was extensive in three of them. The fifth patient (2) showed multiple granulomas with giant cells throughout his liver, although no organisms were discovered. The intestinal parasites most commonly found were *H. nana* (in four patients) and *T. trichiura* (in three patients). Two patients showed heavy infestation with *Ascaris lumbricoides.* Light infestations with *Entamoeba histolytica, Giardia lamblia* and *Necator americanus* were manifested in one patient.

Serum Chemistry.

Hyperglobulinemia was present in four patients (1, 3, 4 and 5), and elevation of thymol turbidity and cephalin flocculation was present in the three patients who exhibited the greatest hyperglobulinemia (1, 4 and 5). The maximum thymol turbidity to be determined was a value of 12 in patients 1 and 5, who also showed the maximum cephalin flocculation with a four plus reaction.

Serum cholesterol examinations revealed mild or transient abnormalities in three patients (1, 2 and 3), with the minimum serum cholesterol value of 49 mg per 100 ml in patient 1. Triglycerides, phospholipides and free cholesterol values were either slightly depressed or at the lower margin of normal in these patients.

Depressions to low or slightly subnormal levels were found in serum Vitamin A and carotene determinations in patient 1; in patients 2 and 3 normal values were found. BSP retention was 12 percent on one occasion in patient 5. Serum transaminase values were elevated during the febrile reaction of patient 3 (maximum SGOT: 71, maximum SGPT: 78). In contrast, serum transaminase was normal in the other four patients.

Prothrombin time was elevated to 17 seconds in patient 1, compared with a control value of 13 seconds. Intravenous injections of vitamin K_1 oxide (Mephyton®) produced only slight improvement. Patient 1 manifested gross melena for three days following jejunal biopsy with a Crosby capsule. Although his platelet count was reduced to 120,000, and prothrombin time was 17 seconds, his coagulation time in vitro was normal. A definite cause for melena was never established.

Alkaline phosphatase was within the normal range for adults in all patients except 3, who was pubertal. Patient 3 initially showed an alkaline phosphatase elevation to 42, but during the febrile reaction of Study Period III the level fell to 7. The elevation initially observed in this patient was believed to be a normal value for him resulting from adolescent osteogenesis: the depression to the range of adult normal values was interpreted as a worsening of his condition. This hypothesis was strengthened by a lack of significant alteration of hepatic architecture in the initial liver biopsy, and by the demineralization of the patient's digits which occurred during Study Period III.

Serum iron values were either normal or became normal following oral administration of ferrous salts in all cases except patient 3, who developed a refractory iron deficiency concurrent with his inflammatory reaction during Study Period III. This patient showed a normal iron binding capacity, and no siderophyllin deficiency due to proteinuria. When serum iron did not increase with oral iron therapy, it was apparent that iron absorption was impaired.

Other abnormalities were observed. An abnormal gastrointestinal series was present in two patients. Patient 1 demonstrated indentation of the intestines by enlarged liver and spleen (Fig. 11); patient 4 had *ascaris* worms in his small intestines which were outlined as filling defects (Fig. 66). In biopsies of buccal and jejunal mucosa in patient 1 small numbers of leprosy organisms were observed. Large numbers of non-cultivable acid-fast bacilli were recovered in gastric aspirations in patients 1, 3 and 5. A follow-up study in patient 1 revealed a decrease in the density of organisms in the gastric aspirate during therapy. Aspiration of gastric contents in patient 4 revealed a few colonies of a mycobacterium, scotochromogenic, Runyon group II. One year after the tests were made patient 5 developed a positive aspirate for *M. tuberculosis.*

Some Normal Results.

Clinical indications of secondary amyloidosis were not present in any of the five patients. Mild hypoalbuminemia was initially observed in patients 1 and 4 and proteinuria was observed occasionally in patients 4 and 3. These laboratory tests were not sufficiently abnormal, however, to suggest the presence of amyloidosis. Each biopsy specimen from the five patients was examined for amyloid deposits, using crystal violet stain; none of the 125 specimens showed amyloid.

Gastric analysis was normal in the three patients in whom it was performed, and oral glucose tolerance tests were normal in all five patients. Oral D-xylose administration was followed by normal urinary excretion rates in the three patients in whom this test was performed. Normal values for serum calcium and phosphorus, and normal barium enema examinations were obtained in the five patients. Normal amounts of muscle fibers and fat droplets were present in the feces.

Summary.

The significant abnormal findings in the liver and gastrointestinal tract in all five patients were:

1) abnormal liver histology, with leprosy bacilli present in all of the patients except the one with dimorphous or tuberculoid leprosy. This patient's biopsy revealed granulomas, but no bacilli.
2) large numbers of intestinal parasites.

Two or more patients demonstrated hyperglobulinemia, elevation in the serum thymol turbidity and cephalin flocculation, and leprosy bacilli in gastric aspirates. One patient showed hepatosplenomegaly and a slight prolongation of the prothrombin time. In another patient a transient elevation of BSP retention was observed. One patient revealed a severe iron deficiency anemia. Mild or transient depressions were observed in several patients in serum cholesterol, Vitamin A, carotene and plasma lipids. The patient who showed leprosy bacilli in buccal and jejunal biopsy specimens experienced a diminution in the density of bacilli in gastric aspirates after three months of DDS therapy. The serum bilirubin remained within the normal range in all patients at all times, and amyloidosis was not demonstrable in any patient.

X. RENAL FUNCTION AND PATHOLOGY

Leprosy Bacilli were Present in Two Patients' Kidneys, and Two Other Patients had Proteinuria or Azotemia (Table 11)

Introduction.

The renal lesion of secondary amyloidosis has been the cause of death in many leprosy patients. Powell (1955) and Beddow (1960) reported that renal insufficiency due to secondary amyloidosis has been the major cause of death at the USPHS Hospital for leprosy patients in Carville in recent years. In a report of 50 consecutive autopsies, secondary amyloidosis was found in 46 per cent of cases; in 38 percent of the 50 cases amyloidosis was the cause of death.

Nonspecific nephritis was reported by Kean (1942) as the cause of death in 22 of 103 autopsies in Panamanian leprosy patients, and renal lesions were present in 70 of the 103 cases. The other lesions included 34 cases of acute or chronic nephritis (glomerulonephritis and "type unspecified"). The other types of renal disease were: nephrosclerosis (13), tuberculosis (7), arteriolonephrosclerosis (4), amyloidosis (4), cysts (3), pyelitis (3), calculi (1), and septic infarcts (1).

It is interesting that although nonspecific renal lesions were commonly seen, leprosy bacilli were not found in the renal specimens of these autopsied cases. A renal biopsy in Derbes' (1961) case of diffuse lepromatous leprosy also failed to reveal leprosy bacilli, whereas liver, bone marrow and blood contained large numbers of bacilli. Cases of leprosy of the kidneys are apparently uncommon, although the thorough postmortem studies of Mitsuda revealed a few cases in which leprosy bacilli or lepromas were present in the glomeruli and renal tubules.

Methods.

Examinations of the urine were performed at regular intervals, usually weekly, on the patients in the present series. The specimens were examined for specific gravity, color and turbidity, pH, the presence of reducing substances, protein, acetone, and microscopic abnormalities. Blood urea nitrogen specimens were obtained from each patient during each study period. In the majority of the patients, serial BUN determinations were performed, increasing in frequency during periods of increased illness or fever. Serum creatinine and creatinine clearance determinations were also performed in each patient during each study period. The creatinine clearance measurements were based upon 24-hour urine collections. Urinary protein was evaluated quantitatively in each patient by 24-hour collections and by routine qualitative tests performed as a part of urinalysis. Renal concentrating power was measured by determinations of specific gravity using the Fishberg test, performed during each study period on each patient; repeated measurements were obtained for patient 3 when his renal function was found to be decreasing.

The right kidney of each patient was examined through the surgical incision performed to obtain the renal biopsy. At this time, a specimen of Gerota's perirenal fascia was obtained. The specimens were stained with hematoxylin and eosin, Fite, Ziehl-Nielsen and crystal violet stains. Each specimen was cultured for common pathogenic bacteria, *Mycobacterium tuberculosis* and fungi.

The urine from each patient was concentrated by centrifugation and cultured for tuberculosis. In most cases the specimens were first-voided morning specimens, although on many occasions 24-hour collections were used as a result of the difficulty of patient 1 in voiding more than once daily.

Cultures for bacteria and fungi were performed on each patient's urine, and were repeated during periods of fever and/or observation of leukocytes in the urinary sediment.

Other tests performed on some of the patients were: intravenous pyelogram (patients 4 and 5), serum uric acid (patients 1, 2 and 3), serum calcium and phosphorous (all patients). Also measured in the urine of these patients were the following substances: corticosteroids (all patients, see Table 12), urobilinogen (all patients, see Table 15), and hydroxyproline (patients 1 and 2, see Table 15).

Results.

Abnormalities of renal function were detected in three of the five patients, but only one patient showed persistent, significant abnormalities. Patient 3 had demonstrated normal renal function during Study Periods I and II, but developed impaired function during the febrile reaction of Study Period III. His renal function continued to worsen even after the fever had subsided. The functional impairment in this patient was confirmed by several parameters measured on several occasions. The BUN increased to a maximum of 25, the serum creatinine to 1.5 and uric acid to 4.2 mg percent. Excretion of PSP fell to 34 percent in two hours, and creatinine clearance fell to 45 ml per min. Urinary concentrating power diminished; the maximum specific gravity became 1.016. Proteinuria was observed, and the mean value of protein excretion measured over a 14-day period was 0.5 gm per day, with a maximum value of 0.8 gm per day. The urinary sediment showed white cells and casts intermittently during Study Period III, with a maximum excretion of 30 leukocytes and three hyaline or granular casts per high power field. In two other patients (4 and 5), intermittent proteinuria of a mild degree was observed.

The renal biopsy specimens from patients 1 and 5 showed leprosy bacilli in the glomeruli, in endothelial cells. The percentage of glomeruli which contained bacilli was greater in Patient 1 (who also showed bacilli in his peripheral venous blood) than in patient 5. In patient 1 approximately 25 percent of the glomeruli were involved, whereas in patient 5, only 10 percent of the glomeruli contained bacilli. In the involved glomeruli of patient 1 the number of bacilli was greater than in patient 5 – so much greater, in fact, that an exact count could not be performed. In patient 5, by contrast, the organisms were widely scattered in small groups.

Acid-fast bacilli were not seen in the kidneys of any of the five patients except in glomeruli: none of the patients showed acid-fast bacilli in the urine, although small numbers of acid-fast bacilli were seen in the Gerota's fascia of patient 1.

All of the histologic studies for amyloidosis were negative. None of the urine specimens revealed growth of *M. tuberculosis.* The mild urinary tract infections with gram negative organisms which developed postoperatively in patients 1, 2 and 5 responded promptly to chemotherapy with tetracycline or sulfisoxzole. Pathogenic fungi were not recovered from the urine of any patient.

Significance of the Studies.

The results of these studies clearly indicate that although renal abnormalities are not always present in leprosy, significant abnormalities may be detected in some patients. Great concern was expressed concerning proteinuria and diminished clearance in patient 3 when he did not improve after his febrile reaction had subsided. The progressive abnormality was so ominous that his DPT dosage was reduced from 1.5 gm per day to 0.5 gm per day in view of DPT toxicity as a possible cause. When his abnormalities were first observed prior to DPT therapy they were believed to be due to increased glomerular permeability. However, as the edema of his subcutaneous tissues diminished and liver function improved, renal function remained depressed.

We believed that DPT may have contributed to the abnormality in renal function in patient 3. This suggests that careful studies of the effect of DPT on renal function should be carried out in patients who receive this drug. Measurements of BUN and serum creatinine may not be sufficient to detect mild or early abnormalities; the additional tests described above should also be carried out.

The proteinuria discovered in patients 4 and 5 on intermittent occasions cannot be explained at the present time. It is possible that such small amounts of protein might have been reported as the result of laboratory error, especially since the finding occurred only once in patient 5. Orthostatic albuminuria also probably occurs occasionally in leprosy, as it does in normal people.

It was especially interesting that the patient with the most extensive involvement of the kidneys and perirenal area by leprosy bacilli showed no abnormalities in renal function.

XI. ADRENAL FUNCTION

Adrenal Insufficiency was Suspected in Three Cases, but Proof was Difficult to Obtain (Tables 12 and 13)

Extensive abnormalities of the adrenal gland have been reported in some cases of leprosy at autopsy. The abnormalities most commonly reported have been lepromas, amyloidosis and atrophy. In Mitsuda's experience (1937) with 1000 autopsies in leprosy patients, the macroscopic lesions of leprosy were predominantly present in four organs in addition to the skin: liver, spleen, adrenals and testicles. Black (1938) reported 5 out of 46 autopsies showed lepromas of the adrenals and Fite (1943) commented that the "adrenal gland not infrequently shows small miliary leprous foci." In autopsied leprosy cases, Grabstald and Swan (1951) found adrenal amyloidosis in "all subjects whose testes exhibited interstitial cells in larger than normal numbers." On the other hand, a high incidence of leprosy of the adrenal glands is not universally reported, for Kean (1942) found adrenal disease in only nine of his 103 leprosy autopsies, the abnormalities being due to leprosy, tuberculosis amyloidosis, and adrenal atrophy.

No reports are known in which abnormalities in adrenal function are well documented in patients with leprosy. However, when extensive anatomical destruction is present, functional impairment might be observed if appropriate tests are performed.

Adrenal function was measured in our five patients by baseline 24-hour urine collections for 17 hydroxy corticosteroids (17OHCS) and 17 keto steroids (17KS). These studies were followed by ACTH tests, in which measurements were made of plasma corticoids and urinary 17OHCS, 17KS and creatinine. Each patient was also tested with SU4885 (Metopirone®; metyrapone USP CIBA) to evaluate pituitary secretion of ACTH.

Normal results in this laboratory, for men aged 14 to 30, were:

urinary 17OHCS	4–14 mg/24 hours
urinary 17KS	10–24 mg/24 hours
plasma corticoids	5–20 μgm/100 ml

The assessment of data is based on 75 specimens for 17OHCS, 70 specimens for 17KS, and 21 specimens for plasma corticoids in the five patients tested. The ACTH tests include 15 intravenous tests and one intramuscular test in which ACTH was given for seven days. All determinations were performed in duplicate. All of the data are summarized in Tables 12 and 13.

17OHCS Excretion and Plasma Corticoids.

The average basal excretion of urinary 17OHCS was normal in each case, but only patients 4 and 5 showed a consistently normal increase in excretion of 17OHCS following stimulation by ACTH and SU4885. Abnormally low values for urinary 17OHCS and plasma corticoids were found on many occasions from patients 1, 2, 3 and 4. The mean basal 17OHCS excretion in the five patients was 6.5 (5.3–8.3), and the mean value with stimulation was 14.1 (9.7–21.3). Thirty-nine specimens were analyzed for creatinine, also. The mean creatinine excretion was 890 mg per 24 hours. Mean values for the individual patients varied from 672–1330 mg per 24 hours, which were normal for their body weights. Adrenal insufficiency was strongly suspected in patients 1, 2 and 3.

Patient 1 showed a normal increase in circulating plasma corticoids in only one of seven ACTH tests. His normal ACTH test was observed after five months of DDS therapy, when he was clinically improved. Of a total of twenty-two 24-hour urine collections analyzed for 17OHCS, twelve were obtained from this patient during ACTH administration and two during SU4885. On only four of the twenty-two 17OHCS collections was steroid excretion greater than the range of values for normal basal output. Six 24-hour urine collections from patient 1 contained less than 4 mg per 24 hours, and the maximum value on the day of an ACTH test was only 21.5 mg per 24 hours.

In studies of patient 2, 2 out of 10 specimens of 24-hour 17OHCS excretion were subnormal. The response to ACTH and SU4885 in this patient may have been normal, since plasma corticoids increased promptly during the two ACTH tests, and urinary excretion of 17OHCS rose to greater than the normal range during one of the three periods of adrenal stimulation. Nevertheless, it should be emphasized that although an increase in 17OHCS excretion was observed following both ACTH and SU4885 in patient 2, only one result in three tests showed a distinct increase. On this occasion the 17OHCS excretion increased to 14.3 mg, which is a mere 0.3 mg above normal basal output.

Patient 3 showed a normal ACTH test during his early hospitalization (Study Period I), but at the end of Study Period II he was found to have no increase in plasma corticoids when ACTH was administered. Before the ACTH test could be repeated to check this unexpected finding, he developed the severe febrile reaction described above. He was eventually treated with prednisone, followed by a test with ACTH intramuscularly for one week, and no increase in plasma corticoids developed. Several weeks after steroids had been discontinued, ACTH (40 units intravenously) was administered, and a small rise in plasma corticoids was finally observed.

17KS Excretion.

Urinary excretion of 17KS was significantly less than normal in three (1, 2, 3) of the five patients, somewhat less than normal in one patient (5), and possibly decreased in the fifth patient (4). In general, a remarkably low pattern of 17KS excretion was seen in the five young men.

As a whole, the group of five patients produced low levels of 17KS excretion in 50 out of 70 collections. Not a single value was greater than normal, even in 18 patient-days of ACTH stimulation and six patient-days of SU4885 stimulation. The excretion ranged as low as 0.3–3.3 mg per 24 hours in cases 1, 2, 3 and 4. The mean basal excretion of 17KS was 7.2 (3.8–9.9) and with stimulation rose to 9.8 (8.0–12.2).

In cases 1 and 4, who had severe lepromatous orchitis, 17 out of 26 basal collections were below normal, being less than 10 mg per 24 hours, and in these two patients the depression of 17KS output was probably related to testicular destruction. Basal excretion and three periods of ACTH or SU4885 stimulation all failed to produce 17KS levels up to the normal range in patient 5, who had moderately severe leprous orchitis. Even in patients 2 and 3, who demonstrated relatively normal testicular histology, 17KS excretion was usually low. In patients 2 and 3, and possibly in all five cases, the low 17KS excretion may have been a manifestation of some degree of adrenal insufficiency.

Analysis of the Data, and Some Additional Reflections.

Consideration of adrenal pathology in leprosy, especially in autopsied cases, must take into account the high incidence of tuberculosis which is known to occur in patients with leprosy in underdeveloped areas of the world. Since tuberculosis of the adrenal glands is a common cause of adrenal insufficiency, reported cases of "leprosy" of the adrenals require careful scrutiny before acceptance. A "negative" culture for tuberculosis may be viewed with suspicion if the patient has recently received antitubercular therapy.

None of the patients in the present report had positive cultures for tuberculosis, and antituberculosis therapy was not administered to them. Patient 5 developed tuberculosis one year later, and was treated for it with INH and PAS. Since patient 5 showed normal responses to ACTH and SU4885, the development of tuberculosis in this case was not considered relevant to the discussion of adrenal insufficiency.

The SU4885 (Metopirone, metyrapone) test is performed to evaluate pituitary secretion of ACTH. SU4885 inhibits 11-beta-hydroxylation, causing a decrease in cortisol biosynthesis. This leads to increased pituitary secretion of ACTH and increased amounts of precursor metabolites, measured as 17OHCS and 17KS. Normal adrenal function is required for evaluation of pituitary ACTH secretion.

In at least three of the five cases presented in this report adrenal function was impaired or questionable. Yet when these patients received SU4885 none of them became ill — a phenomenon that has been observed in patients with several adrenal insufficiency. In all five, the ACTH and SU4885 tests gave essentially the same results, which indicates there was no demonstrable difference in activity between endogenous and exogenous ACTH in these patients and that no pituitary dysfunction is evident.

A final conclusion cannot be reached concerning the quality of adrenal function in these five young men with leprosy. Time was too short, and the state of the disease too variable, to allow for performance of definitive studies. Furthermore, repeated infusions of ACTH seemed unwarranted in testing patients with disseminated mycobacterial disease. Only a tentative conclusion, then, is presented.

Strong suggestive evidence has been presented for a diagnosis of partial adrenal insufficiency in patient 1 (which improved with therapy), in patient 2, and, during part of his hospitalization, in patient 3. The remarkably low values of 17KS excretion which were observed suggest that testicular androgen synthesis was diminished in three cases, and possibly in all five. The effects of adrenal and testicular hypofunction were often superimposed and indistinguishable.

XII. REPRODUCTIVE FUNCTION

Testicular Destruction to a Remarkable Degree is Discovered Early in Leprosy (Table 14)

A high incidence of testicular infection in leprosy was pointed out by Mitsuda (1952) and Fite (1943). Kean's series of 103 leprosy autopsies included five cases of leprosy of the testicles, three of the epididymis, and one each of leprosy of the prostate and penis. Thirty cases of fibrosis, atrophy or chronic inflammation of the testicles were also attributed to previous infection with leprosy.

The problem of leprous orchitis, and its association with gynecomastia, was studied by Job (1961). In 21 leprous patients with gynecomastia, he found that the testicular Leydig cells were hypertrophied (enlarged), clumped, and present in increased numbers. On the other hand, in the cases without gynecomastia, the Leydig cells were normal, reduced in number, or absent. Acid-fast bacilli were seen in the testicles of all lepromatous cases. 17KS excretion was low in the six patients studied, four of whom had gynecomastia.

Since the Leydig cells are assumed to be the site of testosterone production in the testicles, decreased production of testosterone metabolites (17KS) in patients with hypertrophy of Leydig cells appears to be paradoxical. This paradox was not fully explained by Job. He suggested that these patients had an acquired Kleinfelter-like syndrome, with atrophy of the seminiferous tubules, stimulation of gonadotrophins, and increased production of estrogens by the Leydig cells. Decreased inactivation of estrogens in the leprous liver was postulated as the final step in production of gynecomastia.

Grabstald and Swan studied gynecomastia and testicular atrophy in 179 patients with leprosy. Twenty-eight percent of testicles measured were atrophic (less than 2.0 x 3.0 cm), and 19 percent of the patients had gynecomastia. Three phases in leprosy of the testicles were recognized: vascular phase (active leprous orchitis), interstitial cell phase (with fibrosis of seminiferous tubules), and obliterative phase (complete fibrosis). In the second phase clumping of interstitial cells was observed, but true interstitial cell hyperplasia appeared to be doubtful. Two patients (one with gynecomastia) showed normal 17KS and elevated urinary gonadotrophins.

Grabstald and Swan concluded that leprous orchitis was frequent, occurring in every patient whose testicles were examined microscopically, and that many patients who had testis atrophy did not also have gynecomastia. They suggested that leprosy patients with testicular atrophy and gynecomastia had hypergonadotrophic eunuchoidism — that this was one of the few disease entities in the group described by Kleinfelter et al. whose etiology was known.

We are unaware of any previous studies of testicular anatomy and function in young men with early leprosy infections. The present studies eliminate the possible effects of antileprosy therapy on reproductive function, since the majority of the tests in this report were performed before therapy was instituted.

The following studies were carried out in all five patients to the extent possible in each case: semen or prostatic fluid examination, open biopsies, measurements and photographs of testicles, seminal vesiculograms, urinary chorionic gonadotrophin (CGT) measurements, urinary 17KS measurements. A careful history of sexual behavior and capacity was recorded. Results of additional tests performed in one or more patients are recorded elsewhere in this report; the reader's attention is called to these studies as they relate to reproductive function: prostatic biopsies, examination of scrotal and prepuce histology, biopsy of enlarged breast tissue, examination of breast discharge for leprosy bacilli, and cystometrogram.

Seminal emission was obtained from three of the five patients, and abnormalities were observed in two of the three. Patient 1 produced only 0.5 ml of semen, an unusually viscid specimen containing many acid-fast bacilli. No sperm were present. In the seminal emission from patient 3 (also of small volume — 0.7 ml), 17 percent of the sperm present showed abnormal morphology when examined by the Papanikolau technique. This specimen exhibited normal motility, viscosity and density (73,000,000 per ml) of sperm. Normal semen was produced by patient 4. One patient (2) was unable to ejaculate for the test, probably because of psychological inhibition; he stated that he ejaculated normally at other times. Patient 5 was unable to sustain an erection or ejaculation because of severe lepromatous balanoposthitis.

Four of the patients revealed abnormalities of the testicles; the only patient with normal testicles was the 14-year-old boy with indeterminate leprosy (patient 3). Total destruction of spermatogenesis, atrophy, and a heavy density of leprosy bacilli were found in patient 1. A photograph of these testicles is shown in Fig. 86. Slight testicular enlargement was present in patient 2, as illustrated in Fig. 87. This patient had fibrosis and tubular atrophy, with a decrease in spermatogenesis. Patients 4 and 5 had grossly normal testicles, but on histologic examination both revealed acid-fast bacilli, inflammation and fibrosis.

The histopathology in the leprosy patients is illustrated in photomicrographs which accompany this report. Lepromatous testicles are shown in Figs. 20, 68, 79 and 80. The enlarged, fibrotic and partially destroyed testicle of patient 2 is shown in Fig. 40.

The interstitial cells were absent in patient 1 (Fig. 20), decreased in patients 2 (Fig. 40) and 4 (Fig. 68), and slightly decreased in patient 5 (Fig. 79). Mild chronic gynecomastia was present in patient 1 (Fig. 6). Acute, temporary gynecomastia with bacilli in nipple secretions was observed in patient 4. Our small series of patients with early leprosy did not provide either confirmation or rebuttal of Job's hypotheses.

Severe lepromatous infiltration of the scrotum in patient 1 is illustrated in Figs. 14 and 15, and a similar lesion of the foreskin in patient 5 is shown in Figs. 76 and 77. The discovery of leprosy organisms in the prostate of patient 1 is depicted in Fig. 22.

The urinary gonadotrophin production of patient 1 was found to be increased to the eunuchoid range (500 mouse units), and slight elevation was present in the gonadotrophin excretion in patient 2. These findings are similar to those reported by Martin (1968), who found elevated gonadotrophins and decreased plasma testosterone levels in lepromatous males with gynecomastia and testicular atrophy.

Seminal vesiculograms were performed in the operating room in all patients. In three cases distinctly abnormal findings were recorded which demonstrated delayed emptying of the seminal vesicles. These patients (2, 4 and 5) were the only individuals among the five who had had intercourse, and all three had had gonorrhea. The delayed emptying of the seminal vesicles was probably not the result of infection with leprosy but was significant as an additional burden on reproductive function. Radiologic examples of partially obstructed seminal vesical outflow are shown in Figs. 32 and 82.

Patient 4 was the only case who reported frequent sexual intercourse prior to his admission to the Clinical Center. This patient demonstrated the highest urinary 17KS excretion of the five. The others, for psychological and physical reasons, no longer established close relationships with women. Two patients (2 and 5), who reported regular sexual relations prior to the development of symptoms of leprosy, had been separated from their paramours for many months. Patient 5 was in fact the father of two children, whom he had not seen for four years.

Through regular opportunities given them to talk with a psychiatric social worker, the five patients frequently discussed their fears and desires concerning sex. Feelings of inadequacy, physical deformity, competition, loneliness, and curiosity about women's attitudes toward them were repeatedly expressed. They were anxious about their desires to walk, talk, and dance with the American girls whom they met at the Clinical Center; "pin-up girls" were highly prized decorations in their rooms. But they understood that permission to stay in the United States depended on their obeying hospital rules, and they agreed to avoid physical contact with non-infected patients and laymen. This agreement undoubtedly must have contributed to their anxiety, as did their unfamiliarity with American customs and language. On the other hand, these patients had the advantage of being members of a group which shared experiences and had group defenses. In contrast to many patients at the Center, they exhibited a relative lack of deformity of surface features, and this made their social mobility easier. The hospital encouraged them in this by giving them a small allowance to spend each week.

In summary, four of the five patients demonstrated a remarkably severe degree of disease of the genitalia, and one patient, at age 17, was undoubtedly already rendered permanently sterile by leprosy. All five patients showed abnormalities in either seminal emission or testicular structure. Androgen production, as measured by urinary 17KS excretion, was definitely low in three patients, and was probably impaired in the other two. All patients revealed a deep-seated feeling of sexual inadequacy; their impulsive projection into heterosexual activities alternated with periods of self-conscious withdrawal from feminine companionship.

CONCLUSION

> "Why don't you rest, Father Damien," one of his parishioners asked.
> "Rest?" he retorted, "it's no time to rest now, when there is so much left to do and my time is so short!"
>
> John Farrow, *Damien the Leper*

Five young men with newly-diagnosed, untreated leprosy were studied for periods of three to nine months at the Clinical Center, National Institutes of Health. The studies in each case were performed in a prospective manner, comparable in each patient. The purpose of the investigation was to add to the existing body of information concerning the natural history of leprosy, and to serve as a baseline for a study of the chemotherapy of this disease.

Following a period of observation for two to three months, the patients were treated with one or more chemotherapeutic agents. The drugs used were DDS (diaminodiphenyl sulfone), DPT (diphenyl thiourea), and/or B-663 (rimizine dye derivative). The classification of the type of leprosy exhibited by these patients was, at the time of their admission to the Center: lepromatous (three patients), dimorphous (one patient), and indeterminate (one patient).

The studies performed were classified into several major areas of research: 1) skin and neuromuscular, 2) bacteriology and pathology, 3) immunology, 4) ophthalmology, 5) hematology, 6) gastrointestinal and 7) adrenal-genito-urinary.

The examinations of the skin, nervous system and muscular function were useful in classifying and in following the progress of leprosy and of therapy. All patients exhibited abnormalities in each of these systems, of types previously described by other authors.

The bacteriologic studies included examination of 125 tissue specimens with the Fite stain, and 452 preparations of tissue emulsions, body fluids and secretions stained with the Ziehl-Nielsen stain. *Mycobacterium leprae* organisms were recovered from each patient. To rule out the presence of *M. tuberculosis* and other bacteria or fungi, a total of 400 specimens from the five patients were planted on Lowenstein-Jansen, Sabouraud and blood agar. No tubercle bacilli were recovered during the period described in this report, although one patient developed tuberculosis one year later. Only rare colonies of fungi and other bacteria were observed.

Somewhat unexpected findings were the presence of leprosy bacilli in the prostate and jejunem of a patient with diffuse lepromatous leprosy of the Lucio type. Bacilli were observed in the glomeruli in renal biopsies of two lepromatous patients. Leprosy bacilli were found in the liver biopsy of a patient who had the clinical appearance of indeterminate leprosy, and large numbers of leprosy bacilli were present in areas of hepatic necrosis in three lepromatous cases. Leprosy bacilli were recovered from the peripheral blood and semen of a lepromatous patient.

The presence of leprosy bacilli in the sputum, gastric aspirate, skin ulceration and breast discharge from various patients provided new confirmation of the general ubiquity of the bacilli in lepromatous patients. The organisms were not present in skeletal muscle or cerebrospinal fluid in these patients. The morphology of the leprosy bacilli did not appear to vary greatly in each individual patient, regardless of the source of the specimens. A moderate variability in the granularity, size and coloration of the organisms, however, was observed between patients.

The tests of immunologic reactivity in the five patients revealed false positive serologic tests for syphilis in two of the three lepromatous cases; the other nonspecific serologic tests were positive in one patient or another. Lepromin reagent provided a useful, though not perfectly satisfactory, means of classifying the patients. Usefulness of this reagent was limited by the changing degree of reactivity in two patients, and by the borderline size of the nodule (0.3 mm, with granulomatous histology) which developed in one patient. Tuberculin test reactivity was not related to the reactivity to lepromin, in either a positive or negative fashion. All five patients reacted with a positive test to Candidan, Trichophyton or tuberculin. Kveim tests, performed in two patients, were negative.

The five patients showed some degree of abnormality in the serum proteins. The abnormality was of great magnitude, however, only in the patient with diffuse lepromatous leprosy. This patient showed an elevation in total protein, total globulin, gamma globulin, and in IgG, IgA, and IgM fractions. He also showed a low serum albumin level. Elevated globulins and decreased albumin levels were observed in two other patients. The IgM fraction appeared to be increased in four of the five patients. In general, the total globulin and gamma globulin tended to decrease as the patients improved and increase during periods of deterioration. The serum albumin fell to abnormally low levels in one patient during a febrile reaction. The serial measurements of serum proteins and protein fractions, however, were not as useful for quantitation of the patients' status as were bacteriologic studies and measurements of erythrocyte sedimentation rate.

All five patients had significant ophthalmological problems, illustrating the importance of ophthalmologic care for patients with leprosy. In all cases there were problems directly related to leprous infection. One patient showed bacilli in his conjunctival scrapings, one had diminished corneal sensation, and the other three patients demonstrated impaired motion of the eyelids due to leprosy. Chorioretinitis, poor visual acuity, and strabismus were observed in these patients.

Hematologic abnormalities were observed in all patients. The studies performed cast new light on old problems in leprosy and raised new questions. Anemia was observed in all five patients, to a significant degree in three of them. Decreased iron absorption, decreased hematopoesis, and increased hemolysis were demonstrated in various cases. A hemolytic effect of sulfone therapy was suspected but was not proved to be present in any patient.

Of particular interest in one patient were leukopenia, thrombocytopenia, anemia, hepatosplenomegaly and splenic red cell trapping, which were documented with red cell labelled Cr^{51}. Also of interest was an unusual periodic anemia in another patient, associated with erythema nodosum reactions. In the latter patient, each episode of anemia subsided spontaneously with decline of the febrile reactions, and the anemia was demonstrated to be of complex origin. Elevation of the erythrocyte sedimentation rate was observed at one time or another in every patient. This test was the most valuable non-bacteriologic technique for assessing the patient's clinical status.

The gastrointestinal system was studied radiologically, histologically, and functionally. It was generally apparent that the GI system — except for the liver — was remarkably free of disease in these patients. In all liver biopsies, on the other hand, histological abnormalities were found. Four patients showed leprosy bacilli and one revealed widespread granulomatous liver disease. One of the patients was believed to have indeterminate leprosy until bacilli were observed in his liver biopsy. This was believed to be a grave prognostic sign, and he was later reclassified as lepromatous. No previous reports of the performance of a liver biopsy in a patient with indeterminate leprosy are known to exist.

Intestinal parasitism and abnormalities in serum lipids were of interest, but cannot be directly attributed to infection by leprosy. In contrast to findings in patients at the USPHS Hospital at Carville, where amyloidosis is reported to be common in even young people with lepromatous leprosy, amyloidosis was not found in the patients in this series. A finding of interest, although not documented as a part of the gastrointestinal tract studies, was that the density of acid-fast bacilli recoverable from gastric aspirates correlated well with the patients' bacteriologic status during therapy.

The genitourinary and adrenal systems in all of the patients exhibited significant abnormalities. Previous reports indicating that testicular leprosy was common had dealt predominantly with elderly patients who had longstanding leprosy infections. It was surprising and disquieting, therefore, to find abnormalities of the testicles or semen in all five young men in the present study. One patient had apparently been rendered permanently sterile by leprous orchitis at age 17, before he was even known to have leprosy. Two patients had severe leprous orchitis; another exhibited severe testicular fibrosis and atrophy. Understandably, the physical and psychological aspects of genital leprosy were found to be of great importance to the patients themselves. The finding of organisms in renal biopsies from young patients is unique to the present study: collections of leprosy organisms in the kidneys have previously been observed only in postmortem examinations.

It was remarkably difficult to demonstrate normal adrenal function in the five patients in this study. This report concludes with the hypothesis that adrenal cortical function may have been impaired in three of the cases. Abnormally low values for 17OHCS and plasma corticoids were found on many occasions in four patients; only two showed a consistently normal increase in 17OHCS excretion with adrenal stimulation. In the patient with diffuse lepromatous leprosy, adrenal insufficiency was strongly suspected. Urinary excretion of 17KS showed a tendency toward low values in all five patients. This fact was attributed to a combined effect of impaired testicular and adrenal function.

A slow but definite general improvement was observed during therapy in each patient. By contrast, in one case a sudden deterioration occurred following three months of therapy with DDS. This suggests that measurements of slow response to conventional therapy may provide a useful basis for comparison with the effects of more potent chemotherapeutic agents as they become available.

The most promising future areas of clinical research on patients with leprosy appear to include investigation of anemia with radioisotopes and conventional hematologic techniques, assessment of genital and adrenal function, and controlled tests of other chemotherapeutic agents. A severe degree of permanent functional damage had already occurred in the five young men of this study by the time they were first suspected of having leprosy. The most urgent need, then, is earlier diagnosis and prevention of irreversible tissue destruction by providing therapy in the initial stages of the disease. Critically needed are specific skin and serologic tests which would uncover early cases of leprosy.

A POINT OF VIEW

"To thy sickness there shall be no cure . . .
Where thou comest each man shall flee."

The Gods' curse of leprosy
upon Cressida

A Synthesis of the Experimental Results, Clinical Observations and Hypotheses

In this section of the report some of the hypotheses are presented which have been used to organize the program of clinical research in leprosy at the National Institutes of Health. These hypotheses gradually evolved during the year of clinical investigation into the cases of the five leprosy patients. We recognize that some of these hypotheses may eventually be discarded, whereas the truth of others may be proved. The hypotheses are presented simply to stimulate meaningful arguments and productive research in leprosy.

Introduction.

Leprosy is caused by the acid-fast bacillus, *Mycobacterium leprae*. The organism was first seen by Hansen in the early 1870's. It has not yet been successfully cultured in vitro in a cell-free medium. *M. leprae* is fastidious and has a long generation time. Although it has reportedly been difficult to transmit the organism in human experiments, transmission to the mouse foot pad has been achieved by Shepard (1960). Rees (1967) has recently produced generalized lepromatous disease with human leprosy bacilli in irradiated, thymectomized mice. *M. leprae* grows favorably at temperatures below 37.5°C.

Leprosy is probably transmitted by direct inoculation of large numbers of organisms in intimate contact, such as by kissing, or in poor hygienic conditions associated with nasal discharge and sputum, or by inoculation through a broken surface of the skin. Susceptibility to leprosy is greatest in infancy and in association with severe chronic diseases, such as kwashiorkor and malaria. The high incidence in some family groups suggests that a genetic predisposition to leprosy may exist, although this has not been proved.

The predominant occurrence of leprosy in the tropics is probably related more to poor general standards of hygiene than to specific vectors or to association with a specific tropical disease. Leprosy has been endemic in some cold climates — particularly in the Scandinavian countries — within the past 100 years, and there is no reason to believe that it would not reappear in such climates under the proper circumstances. Adults native to non-endemic areas are usually highly resistant to leprosy, although a definite susceptibility exists, as pointed out by Aycock (1947) and Gray (1961), related to duration of exposure, state of general health of the exposed individual, and the density of the inoculation to which he has been exposed.

Judging from previous experience in leprosy hospitals, leprosy is unlikely to develop in medical personnel.

Propositions.

1. Leprosy should be suspected in a patient whenever acid-fast bacilli are recovered which will not grow in culture. (It is recognized, however, that tubercle bacilli may fail to grow in vitro after chemotherapy has been administered.)
2. Leprosy should be suspected in every case of a skin lesion characterized by discoloration and hypesthesia.
3. A diagnosis of leprosy should be considered as doubtful unless acid-fast bacilli can be recovered in biopsy or scrapings *and* an area of cutaneous anesthesia can be demonstrated.
4. Even at the stage of earliest manifestation, leprosy should be viewed as a multi-system disease. It affects the skin and peripheral nervous system, may also invade the oral and nasopharyngeal mucosa, the reticuloendothelial system, (including lymph nodes, liver, bone marrow and circulating blood) and — in male patients — may affect the external genitalia. The only exception to this rule is localized tuberculoid leprosy in which only a single lesion of the skin is detectable.
5. For reasons which are still unknown, leprosy spares the brain, spinal cord, autonomic nervous system, skeletal muscle, heart and lungs in the vast majority of cases.
6. Adrenal cortical dysfunction should be suspected in patients with lepromatous leprosy.
7. Sterility resulting from lepromatous orchitis should be suspected in young men with lepromatous leprosy.

8. Large numbers of leprosy bacilli can be recovered from the sputum, nasal discharge and serous discharges from the skin in untreated young patients with lepromatous leprosy. These body surfaces and secretions should be considered as the most hazardous reservoirs of infected material.
9. Airborne transmission from the upper respiratory tract, and insect vectors, as proposed by McFadzean (1961), should be recognized as possible routes of communicable spread of the disease.
10. Young men with lepromatous leprosy may demonstrate prompt improvement in bacterial status with sulfone therapy. When it is difficult to detect organisms in skin and nasal scrapings, it may be concluded that the hazard of secondary transmission is probably reduced to a negligible level.
11. There is no universal correlation between a patient's appearance and his bacteriologic status. Extensive skin lesions, neuropathy, fever and leonine facies may exist in patients with few leprosy bacteria.
12. Evidence of erythema nodosum or peripheral neuropathy should suggest the possibility of leprosy in persons who have lived in leprosy endemic areas.
13. The lepromin skin test is a useful means of evaluating improvement in leprosy: when the skin test of a patient with leprosy converts from "negative" to "positive," bacteriologic improvement has probably taken place.
14. Normal adults who have not previously been exposed to leprosy usually show "positive" reactions to lepromin which are clinically indistinguishable from "positive" reactions in leprosy patients. It follows that lepromin skin test is not a useful screening test for the diagnosis of leprosy.
15. Bizarre anemias of complex origin are present in patients with leprosy. Among the causes are: hypersplenism, iron deficiency, spontaneous hemolytic episodes, chronic leprous bacteremia, renal dysfunction, granulomatous and leprous replacement of marrow, intestinal parasites and drug-induced hemolytic anemia.
16. Patients with leprosy may show clinical and bacteriologic improvement when hospitalized and given symptomatic care. The improvement will usually accelerate when sulfone therapy is given. Occasionally disabling complications may occur during therapy although bacteriologic improvement continues.
17. Short courses of steroid therapy may relieve erythema nodosum

reactions in leprosy without necessarily causing demonstrable bacteriologic deterioration.

18. In 1962–63 no satisfactory method of treating acute reactions was available; today's methods are still far from ideal. The report of the use of flufenamic acid by Goodwin in 1968 was encouraging, but controlled studies of many non-steroidal anti-inflammatory agents are urgently needed.

19. An abnormality in serum proteins which is specific for leprosy has not been discovered. Lepromatous leprosy is associated with a variety of nonspecific serological reactions, but no universal serological test for leprosy is known.

20. Delayed hypersensitivity reactions are impaired in most patients with lepromatous leprosy, compared with patients who have tuberculoid leprosy or with normal human beings. It is not known whether impaired reactivity precedes or follows the development of the lepromatous state.

21. At the present time, sulfone derivatives, particularly DDS (diaminodiphenyl sulfone), are the drugs of choice in leprosy. DPT (diphenyl thiourea) is the most useful second drug, to be used in addition to, or instead of DDS, in selected cases.

Leprosy can be effectively studied and treated in a general hospital, in a research hospital, or in a university medical center, if precautions are followed similar to those for active tuberculosis.

APPENDIX

NORMAL VALUES
(Young Male Adult)

Test	*Normal Value or Reaction*
Serum Proteins	
total protein	6.8–8.0 gm/100 ml
albumin	3.5–5.5 gm/100 ml
globulin	1.5–3.4 gm/100 ml
γ-globulin	0.7–1.6 gm/100 ml
Hematology	
hematocrit	38%–54% (average 45%)
hemoglobin	13.5–17.5 gm/100 ml (average 15.5 gm/100 ml)
red blood cell count (RBC)	4.5–6.0 (average 5.0×10^6/cmm)
white blood cell count (WBC)	5,000–10,000/cmm
platelet count	175,000–400,000/cmm
erythrocyte sedimentation rate (ESR)	0–7 mm/hr
red blood cell half life (Cr^{51} $t^{1/2}$)	28 days
blood volume	68–78 ml/kg
red blood cell mass	25–40 ml/kg
reticulocytes	0.5–1.0%
iron, serum	50–150 μgm/100 ml
Liver and Intestinal Function	
cholesterol, serum (total)	110–300 mg/100 ml
cholesterol, serum (free)	35–90 mg/100 ml
triglycerides, plasma	190–420 mg/100 ml
phospholipids, plasma	170–330 mg/100 ml
thymol turbidity, serum	0–5
cephalin flocculation, serum	0 to 1+
phosphatase, alkaline, serum	4–13 KA units
prothrombin time	50–100%
bilirubin, total, serum	0.2–1.0 mg/100 ml
glutamic oxaloacetic transaminase, serum (SGOT)	9–45 units
glutamic pyruvic transaminase, serum (SGPT)	5–35 units
Vitamin A, serum	40–60 μgm/100 ml
carotene, serum	60–368 μgm/100 ml

Test	*Normal Value or Reaction*
Renal Function	
blood urea nitrogen (BUN)	7.0–15.0 mg/100 ml
creatinine, serum	0.8–1.5 mg/100 ml
uric acid, serum	2.5–7.0 mg/100 ml
urine	
creatinine, 24 hours	15–25 mg/kg/24 hours
phenolsulfonphthalein excretion, 2 hours	60–85%
specific gravity (max. & min.)	1.025, 1.004
protein, 24 hours	0–0.05 gm/24 hours
creatinine clearance	140 ml/min
Adrenal – Pituitary – Gonad	
17 hydroxy corticosteroids (17OHCS),urine, 24 hr.	4–14 mg
17 ketosteroids (17KS), urine, 24 hr.	10–24 mg
corticoids, plasma	5–20 μgm/100 ml
ACTH and SU4885 test	17OHCS 15–45 mg/24 hrs 17KS 25–50 mg/24 hrs
semen	
volume/emission	>2.0 ml
sperm	
morphology (% normal)	>90%
count	>25x10^6/ml
motility (%/hour)	>80%
gonadotrophins, urine	<65 mouse units

TABLES

TABLE 1
Associated Investigators
NIH

Clinical Director: Dr. Vernon Knight

Clinical Associates:

Dr. Richard Adler	Dr. Frank Loda
Dr. John Bennett	Dr. John Mulholland
Dr. William T. Butler	Dr. Melvin Rubenstein
Dr. Thomas Cate	Dr. James Smith
Dr. William Fleet	Dr. Benjamin Sturgill

Area of Investigation	*Consultant*	*Special Procedures*
Hematologic	Dr. Wendell Rosse	Cr^{51} studies
Gastrointestinal	Dr. L. Frederick Fenster	Liver biopsies
	Dr. Eliot Weser	Intestinal biopsies
	Dr. Leonard Laster	Serum carotene, Vitamin A, xylose tolerance
		Lipid fractionation
Surgical and genitourinary	Dr. William Kiser	Renal, testicular and prostate biopsies, semen analysis, and seminal vesiculograms
Pathologic	Dr. Louis Thomas	Amyloid stains
	Dr. Alan Rabson	Consultation
	Dr. Chapman Binford	Consultation
Endocrine	Dr. Stanley Korenman Dr. Mortimer Lipsett	Plasma and urine corticosteroids
	Dr. Griff Ross	Urine gonadotrophins
	Dr. Jack Robbins	Thyroid consultation
Bacteriologic	Dr. Young	Special cultivation techniques
	Miss Ada Murphy	AFB smears and cultures
Serological	Dr. John Fahey	Serum protein fractionation
	Dr. Sheldon Wolff & Dr. Jose Uriel	Serum immunoelectrophoresis
	Dr. Joseph Bunim	Bentonite flocculation

	Dr. Robert Carpenter	Fluorescent antinuclear test
Ophthalmological	Dr. John Nicholas	Consultation & AFB smears on conjunctiva
Body metabolism	Dr. Ronald Thompson	Metabolic chamber
Patient care	Dr. C. K. Himmelsbach	Consultation
	Dr. James Doull	Consultation
	Dr. John Hanks	Consultation
	Dr. E. B. Johnwick	Consultation
	Dr. Y. T. Chang	Chemotherapy & tissue culture
	Dr. David Fried	Physical therapy, EMG
	Mrs. Janet Elms	Nursing procedures
	Mrs. Carmen Cabrera	Psychotherapy
	Mr. Arnold Sperling	Patient activities

TABLE 2

Abnormalities of the Skin
in Five Patients with Leprosy, Detected by Physical Examination

	Patient				
	1	2	3	4	5
Initial Classification	Lepromatous, diffuse	Dimorphous	Indeterminate	Lepromatous	Lepromatous (possible dimorphous)
Signs & Symptoms	thickened, diffusely smooth hairless face decreased pubic & axillary hair healed scars & triangular leg lesions enlargement of earlobes and nose anhidrosis of large areas of extremities	macules, with raised erythematous margins, tender & painful atrophy of skin on legs, arms burns and cuts on anesthetic areas enlarged nerves seen on inspection easy bleeding in anesthetic areas anhidrosis of macules & extremities	macules, hypochromic, with partial alopecia of back & buttocks enlargement & erythema of earlobes, slight, with hyperkeratosis alopecia & hypochromic macules anhidrosis of macules and extremities LATER: erythema nodosum, exfoliation, and burns and cuts on anesthetic areas	macules, hyper- and hypochromic, (thighs, forearms & back) erythema nodosum, recurrent, of thighs, arms, eyebrow & trunk enlarged nerves seen on inspection and tiny nodosities of the earlobes LATER: gynecomastia, nipple discharge	macules and nodules, hyperchromic macules, hypochromic Leonine facies, early loss of terminal soft tissue from digits gynecomastia phimosis, severe ulcerations, blisters & calluses of feet enlarged nerves seen on inspection

TABLE 2 (Continued)

	Patient				
	1	2	3	4	5
Total Period of Observation	7 months	7 months	9 months	6 months	3 months
Final Classification	Lepromatous, diffuse	Tuberculoid	Lepromatous	Lepromatous	Lepromatous, nodular

TABLE 3

Neuromuscular Abnormalities in Five Patients with Leprosy

	Patient				
	1	2	3	4	5
Anesthesia and Hypesthesia	of 5th finger, right hand, and of cornea, slight	of lesions & extremities totalling 20–28% of body surface at different times.	of lesions & extremities, totalling 14–50% of body surface at different times.	of lesions & extremities, totalling 20–27% of body surface at different times.	of lesions & extremities, totalling 50–64% of body surface at different times.
Skeletal muscular strength*	decreased, but improved with therapy (87%, increasing to 96.5% of normal in 4 mos.)	decreased, but improved with therapy (85%, increasing to 91% of normal in 4 mos.)	approximately 93.5–100% initially, then decreasing progressively to 72%	normal (100%)	normal (100%)
Electromyogram	normal	very abnormal, but improved after therapy with DDS	Initially, a "mild peripheral neuropathy" was observed	normal	
Nerve Conduction time	normal (right ulnar was not tested)	very slow, but improved after therapy	normal	normal	

TABLE 3 (Continued)

	Patient				
	1	2	3	4	5
Nerve enlargement & tenderness	none	ulnar, median, peroneal, posterior auricular, sural, spermatic (bilateral)	ulnar (bilateral)	ulnar peroneal (bilateral)	ulnar peroneal (bilateral)
Other abnormalities	cystometrogram, neuropathic (no effective contractions with 400 ml)	lagophthalmos, severe	lagophthalmos, mild	—	exotropia, bilateral, moderately severe

* Skeletal muscular strength (SMS) is the ratio of observed strength (OS) to normal strength (NS)
The strength in each muscle or muscle group was evaluated qualitatively
Normal strength (NS) was defined as 5 on a semi-quantitative scale
Observed strength (OS) was evaluated on a scale of 0–5

Normal = 5	Poor = 2
Good = 4	Trace = 1
Fair = 3	Zero = 0

$$SMS = \frac{\Sigma OS}{\Sigma NS} \times 100$$

See text (Discussion, Part II) for example

TABLE 4

Bacteriology and Pathology
Mean Density* of Acid-Fast Bacilli in Specimens
Obtained From Five Leprosy Patients at Different Periods in Their Illnesses

		Patient									
		1		2		3		4		5	
Specimens	Study Period**	Density	Specimens	Density	Specimens	Density	Specimens	Density	Specimens	Density	Specimens
Nasal mucosa	I	4	(3)	0***	(3)	1	(4)	3	(6)	4	(6)
	II	4	(8)	0	(8)	3	(4)	3	(6)		
	III					1	(8)				
Skin (ear, eyebrow, extremities, trunk)	I	3	(9)	1***	(9)	1	(11)	2	(19)	2	(26)
	II	3	(30)	0	(20)	2	(12)	1	(15)		
	III					1	(27)				
Skin (scalp, axilla, pubis)	I	—		—		—		—		0	(2)
	II	2	(3)	0	(3)	1	(3)	0	(3)		
	III					—					
Lymph nodes	I	4	(1)	0	(1)	3	(1)	4	(2)	4	(3)
	II	4	(1)	—		—		4	(1)		
	III					2	(2)				
Liver	I	4	(1)	0	(1)	3	(1)	4	(1)	4	(1)
	II	—		—		4	(1)	—			
	III					—					
Blood	I	2	(14)	0	(3)	0	(4)	0	(5)	—	
	II	0	(5)	0	(3)	—		—			
	III					0	(1)				

TABLE 4 (Continued)

		Patient									
		1		2		3		4		5	
Specimens	Study Period**	Density	Specimens	Density	Specimens	Density	Specimens	Density	Specimens	Density	Specimens
Sputum	I	2	(2)	0	(5)	0	(2)	4	(2)	unobtainable	
	II	0	(2)	0	(3)	—		—			
	III					0	(1)				
Gastric washings	I	3	(1)	0	(3)	0	(3)	4	(2)	4	(2)
	II	1	(1)	0	(1)	—		—			
	III					—					
Jejunem	I	—		—		—		—		0	(2)
	II	1	(1)	0	(1)	0	(1)	0	(1)		
	III					—					
Semen	I	3	(1)	unobtainable		0	(1)	0	(1)	unobtainable	
	II	0	(1)	unobtainable		—		—			
	III					0	(1)				
Bone marrow	I	3	(2)	0	(2)	0	(1)	1	(1)	1	(1)
	II	4	(1)	1	(2)	—		—			
	III					1	(2)				
Subcutaneous fat (deep)	I	4	(1)	0	(1)	0	(1)	0	(1)	0	(1)
	II	—		—		—		—		—	
	III					—					
Gerota's fat	I	1	(1)	0	(1)	0	(1)	0	(1)	0	(1)
	II	—		—		—		—		—	
	III					—					

TABLE 4 (Continued)

Specimens	Study Period**	Patient 1 Density	Patient 1 Specimens	Patient 2 Density	Patient 2 Specimens	Patient 3 Density	Patient 3 Specimens	Patient 4 Density	Patient 4 Specimens	Patient 5 Density	Patient 5 Specimens
Testicles	I	4	(1)	0	(1)	0	(1)	3	(2)	4	(2)
Ulceration drainage	I	4	(1)	none present		none present		none present		—	
Buccal mucosa	I	1	(1)	0	(1)	0	(1)	0	(1)	0	(1)
Hydrocele fluid	I	1	(1)	0	(1)	none present		none present		none present	
Kidney	I	1	(1)	0	(1)	0	(1)	0	(1)	1	(1)
Prostate	I	1	(1)	0	(1)	0	(1)	0	(1)	0	(1)
Prostatic discharge	I	none present		none present		none present		none present		3	(1)
Cerebro-spinal fluid	I	—		—		—		0	(1)	0	(1)
	II	0	(1)	0	(1)	0	(1)				
	III					—					
Urine	I	0	(5)	0	(7)	0	(5)	0	(3)		
	II	0	(4)	0	(4)	—	—	—			
	III					—				0	(2)
Feces	I	0	(1)	1	(5)	—		0	(2)	—	

TABLE 4 (Continued)

		Patient									
		1		2		3		4		5	
Specimens	Study Period**	Density	Specimens	Density	Specimens	Density	Specimens	Density	Specimens	Density	Specimens
Feces	II	0	(3)	0	(1)	0	(1)	—			
	III					0	(1)				
Muscle (latissimus dorsi)	I	0	(1)	0	(1)	0	(1)	0	(1)	0	(1)
Nerve (spermatic)	I	—		0	(1)	—		—		—	
Fascia, spermatic	I	4	(1)	—		—		3	(1)	—	
Rectal mucosa	I	—		—		—		0	(1)		
Breast	I	—		—		—		2	(1)	—	
Breast discharge	I	none present		none present		none present		2	(2)	none present	
	II	"		"		"		2	(2)	"	
Ascaris, recovered from pt.	I	none present		none present		none present		—		rod-shaped acid-fast structures in ovary	

TABLE 4 (Continued)

Specimens	Study Period**	Patient 1 Density	Patient 1 Specimens	Patient 2 Density	Patient 2 Specimens	Patient 3 Density	Patient 3 Specimens	Patient 4 Density	Patient 4 Specimens	Patient 5 Density	Patient 5 Specimens
Conjunctival scrapings		0	(1)	0	(1)	0	(1)	0	(1)	present	(1)

* Definition of bacterial density in smears prepared from tissue emulsions and fluid specimens:

Density

4 More than 1 globus or 100 free bacilli present per 100 oil immersion fields (OIF)
3 1 globus per 100–500 OIF, or 50–100 free bacilli seen per 100 OIF
2 No globi present, but 25–50 bacilli seen per 100 OIF
1 1–25 free bacilli per 100 OIF

When more than one specimen was obtained in any Study Period, estimation of the density of the separate specimens are made, and the Mean Density derived from these estimations.

** Definition of Study Periods

I Immediately prior to institution of anti-leprosy chemotherapy. Patients 1, 2 and 3 were studied for two consecutive months; Patients 4 and 5 were studied for three consecutive months.

II The first few months of sulfone therapy. Patients 1 and 2 were studied for five consecutive months; patients 3 and 4 were studied for three consecutive months. Patient 4 also received intermittent therapy with B663 during this period. (Patient 5 had received only one month of therapy with B663 at the time this report was prepared.)

III A "reactive" period in the course of patient 3, which followed Period II, and which lasted for four months. During this time the patient suffered from fever, exfoliative dermatitis and peripheral neuritis, and his treatment was changed from diaminodiphenyl sulfone (DDS) to diphenyl thiourea (DPT) and prednisone.

*** Additional specimens of nasal mucosa and skin scrapings taken at the Centro Dermatologico Pascua two months prior to arrival at the NIH Clinical Center were "positive" for acid-fast bacilli.

TABLE 5

Skin Tests

Performed upon Five Leprosy Patients Before and After Therapy

Test	Study Period**	Patient 1	2	3	4	5
Lepromin 4 hour (Medina)	I	positive (necrosis)	negative	negative	negative	negative
	II	negative	negative	negative	—	
Lepromin 12–36 hour (Fernandez)	I	negative	not recorded	not recorded	positive 8mm	negative
	II	negative	negative	positive 5mm	—	
Lepromin 21 days (Mitsuda)	I	negative	negative	negative	negative	negative
	II	negative	positve 5 mm	± 3mm	—	
Tuberculin (PPD)	I	negative (2nd strength)	positive 10mm (2nd strength)	negative	positive 50mm Intermediate strength)	positive 12mm (0.05 1st strength)
	II	negative (2nd strength)	negative	negative	positive 15mm (0.05 1st strength)	
Candidan (1:30)	I	negative	positive 10mm	positive 6mm	negative	positive 15mm
	II	negative	—	—	—	
Trychophyton (1:30)	I	negative	positive 10mm	positive 6mm	positive 6mm	—
	II	negative	—	—	—	

TABLE 5 (Continued)

Test	Study Period**	Patient 1	2	3	4	5
Histoplasmin	I	negative	negative	negative	negative	positive 10mm
	II	negative	—	negative	—	
Blastomycin	I	negative	negative	negative	negative	negative
	II	negative	—	negative	—	
Coccidiomycin	I	negative	negative	negative	negative	negative
	II	negative	—	negative	—	
Kveim antigen	I	—	—	—	negative	negative
	II	—	—	—	—	

** Study Period: See corresponding footnote for Table 4.

TABLE 6

Serological Tests
in Five Leprosy Patients

Test	Study Period**	Patient 1 Result	Patient 1 Specimens	Patient 2 Result	Patient 2 Specimens	Patient 3 Result	Patient 3 Specimens	Patient 4 Result	Patient 4 Specimens	Patient 5 Result	Patient 5 Specimens
VDRL	I	positive 5x	(7)	0	(1)	0	(1)	weak positive 1x	(3)	0	(1)
	II	positive 3x	(8)	0	(1)	0	(1)	0	(1)		
	III					0	(1)				
Kolmer	I	—		—		—		reactive	(2)	—	
	II	reactive 6x	(8)	—		0	(1)	0	(1)		
	III					0	(1)				
TPI	I	0	(2)	—		—		—		—	
Coombs (direct)	I	positive 2x	(4)	0	(1)	0	(1)	0	(3)	0	(3)
	II	0	(5)	0	(2)	0	(1)	0	(3)		
	III					0	(1)				
C reactive protein	I	2 plus	(2)	0	(1)	0	(1)	4 plus	(3)	1 to 4 plus	(3)
	II	1 to 3 plus	(2)	0	(1)	0	(1)	2 to 4 plus	(3)		
	III					—					

TABLE 6 (Continued)

Test	Study Period**	Patient 1 Result	Patient 1 Specimens	Patient 2 Result	Patient 2 Specimens	Patient 3 Result	Patient 3 Specimens	Patient 4 Result	Patient 4 Specimens	Patient 5 Result	Patient 5 Specimens
Anti-streptolysin titer	I	166–500 units	(3)	0	(1)	125 units	(1)	50–125 units	(3)	166–> 500 units	(3)
	II	333 units	(1)	250 units	(1)	166 units	(1)	50–266	(3)		
	III					> 500 units	(1)				
Latex agglutination	I	positive	(1)	0	(1)	0	(1)	—		0	(1)
	II	—		0	(1)	—		—			
	III					0	(1)				
Heterophile antibody titer	I	positive 1:14	(1)	positive 1:7	(1)	positive 1:7	(1)	—		—	
	II	0	(1)	0	(1)	positive 1:14	(1)	0	(1)		
	III					—					
"Febrile" agglutinins (*Salmonella, Proteus, Brucella, P. tularensis*)	I	0–1:160	(1)	1:20–1:40	(1)	0–1:80	(1)	0 1:400	(1)	0–1:40	(1)
	II	0–1:160	(1)	1:20–1:40	(1)	—		—			
	III					0–1:80	(1)				
Blastomycin C.F.	I	1:16	(1)	0	(1)	0	(1)	—		1:8	(1)
	II	1:32	(1)	—		—		—			
	III					0	(1)				

TABLE 6 (Continued)

Test	Study Period**	Patient 1 Result	Patient 1 Specimens	Patient 2 Result	Patient 2 Specimens	Patient 3 Result	Patient 3 Specimens	Patient 4 Result	Patient 4 Specimens	Patient 5 Result	Patient 5 Specimens
Coccidioidin,	I	0	(1)	0	(1)	0	(1)	—		0	(1)
Histoplasmin	II	0	(1)	—		—		—			
C.F.	III					0	(1)				
Bentonite flocculation	I	1:32 once	(3)	0	(1)	0	(3)	9	(1)	—	
tests	II	—		0	(1)	—		—			
	III					0	(3)				
	I	0	(2)	anti B 1:64	(1)	anti A & B 1:32	(1)	anti A & B 1:32	(2)	anti A & B 1:512	(1)
Iso-hemagglutins	II			anti B 1:64	(1)	—		—			
	III					A 1:128 B 1:256	(1)				
	I	0	(3)	0	(1)	0	(1)	0	(5)	0	(3)
L.E. prep	II	—		0	(1)	—		0	(1)		
	III					—					
Toxoplasmin	I	0	(1)	> 1:1000	(1)	0	(1)	—		—	
dye titer	II	—		—		—		—			
	III					—					

TABLE 6 (Continued)

Test	Study Period**	Patient 1 Result	Patient 1 Specimens	Patient 2 Result	Patient 2 Specimens	Patient 3 Result	Patient 3 Specimens	Patient 4 Result	Patient 4 Specimens	Patient 5 Result	Patient 5 Specimens
Fluorescent antinuclear antibody	I	0	(1)	0	(1)	0	(2)	—		—	
	II	—		—		—		—			
	III					0	(2)				
Anti-thyroglobulin antibody	I	0	(1)	0	(1)	0	(1)	—		—	
Cryoglobulins	I	0	(1)	0	(1)	0	(1)	—		0	(1)
Cold agglutinins	I	0	(1)	0	(1)	0	(1)	0	(1)	0	(1)

**Study Period: See corresponding footnote for Table 4.

TABLE 7
Serum Proteins
Before and After Therapy in Five Leprosy Patients

		Patient									
		1		2		3		4		5	
Serum Protein	Study Period**	Value	Speci-mens	Value	Speci-mens	Value	Speci-mens	Value	Speci-mens	Value	Speci-mens
Total protein	I	9.1	(9)	7.0	(5)	7.6	(5)	6.6	(15)	7.8	(6)
	II	8.7	(18)	6.4	(20)	6.8	(8)	7.3	(14)		
	III					6.6	(17)				
Serum albumin	I	3.2	(9)	4.6	(5)	4.2	(5)	2.9	(15)	3.9	(6)
	II	3.6	(18)	4.2	(20)	3.9	(8)	3.4	(14)		
	III					2.9	(16)				
Serum globulin	I	5.9	(9)	2.6	(5)	3.4	(5)	3.7	(15)	3.9	(6)
	II	5.2	(18)	2.2	(20)	2.9	(8)	3.9	(14)		
	III					3.8	(16)				
γ–globulin	I	4.5	(4)	0.8	(2)	1.5	(1)	1.9	(10)	2.2	(6)
	II	3.6	(11)	0.8	(7)	0.9	(1)	2.0	(11)		
	III					1.8	(15)				

** Study Period See corresponding footnote for Table 4.

TABLE 8

Ophthalmologic Studies in Five Patients with Leprosy

	Patient				
	1	2	3	4	5
Bacteriology (conjunctival scrapings)	negative	negative	negative	negative	positive
Sensation (cornea)	decreased slightly	normal	normal	normal	normal
Visual acuity	normal	O.S. normal O.D. 20/200	O.S. normal O.D. 20/25	normal	normal
Skin and surface	alopecia of eyebrows and eyelashes, thickened conjunctivae	conjunctivitis due to lagophthalmos, initially	conjunctivitis due to lagophthalmos, intermittent	recurrent erythema nodosum of left eyebrow, causing localized alopecia	normal
Symptoms	none	pain due to conjunctivitis, initially severe	pain due to conjunctivitis, temporarily severe	recurrent pain in left upper eyelid, associated with erythema nodosum	dysopia due to exotropia
Corneal nerves (slit-lamp examination)	normal	normal	normal	possibly thickened	possibly thickened
Ophthalmoscopic examination	normal	extensive chorioretinitis, O.D., apparently inactive	possibly a small area of healed chorioretinitis	normal	normal

TABLE 9

Hematologic Abnormalities in Five Patients with Leprosy; Including Studies of Reticuloendothelial System and Bone

		Patient									
		1		2		3		4		5	
Determination	Study Period**	Value (Mean)	Speci-mens	Value (Mean)	Speci-mens	Value (Mean)	Speci-mens	Value (Mean)	Speci-mens	Value (Mean)	Speci-mens
Hematocrit	I	35	(11)	41	(19)	45	(7)	37	(33)	41	(15)
	II	35	(44)	40	(36)	38	(30)	35	(50)		
	III					35	(39)				
Hemoglobin	I	11.9	(11)	13.3	(18)	14.3	(7)	11.6	(27)	12.9	(12)
	II	10.3	(39)	12.4	(45)	11.1	(15)	11.2	(11)		
	III					10.7	(37)				
Red blood cell count	I	4.21	(8)	5.08	(1)	5.22	(2)	4.61	(10)	4.48	(10)
	II	3.90	(8)	3.99	(19)	4.12	(4)	4.36	(4)		
	III					4.60	(13)				
Platelets	I	134	(9)	258	(16)	305	(5)	333	(21)	331	(11)
	II	120	(18)	201	(38)	310	(18)	414	(29)		
	III					355	(35)				
Reticulocytes (%)	I	1.0	(8)	0.6	(1)	1.0	(14)	1.4	(24)	1.4	(8)
	II	2.4	(22)	1.6	(20)	1.4	(15)	1.5	(25)		
	III					1.0	(32)				

TABLE 9 (Continued)

		Patient									
		1		2		3		4		5	
Determination	Study Period**	Value (Mean)	Speci-mens	Value (Mean)	Speci-mens	Value (Mean)	Speci-mens	Value (Mean)	Speci-mens	Value (Mean)	Speci-mens
White blood cell count	I	3600	(11)	4000	(18)	6400	(5)	9400	(32)	8.1	(14)
	II	3900	(46)	3400	(41)	6200	(24)	9600	(43)		
	III					6300	(42)				
Erythrocyte sedimentation rate (Westergren)	I	97	(8)	27	(16)	10	(5)	44	(29)	54	(12)
	II	87	(34)	3	(41)	8	(22)	60	(39)		
	III					33	(37)				
Red blood cell Cr^{51} half life	I							> 28 days	(1)	29 days	(1)
	II	14 days	(1)	18 days	(1)	28 days	(1)	> 28 days	(1)		
Blood volume	I							77.3 ml/kg	(1)	63.1 ml/kg	(1)
	II	80.0 ml/kg	(1)	55.4 ml/kg	(1)	70.0 ml/kg	(1)	80.9 ml/kg	(1)		
Red blood cell volume	I							25.1 ml/kg	(1)	30.8 ml/kg	(1)
	II	24.6 ml/kg	(1)	21.8 ml/kg	(1)	24.5 ml/kg	(1)	25.1 ml/kg	(1)		
Serum iron	I	39	(2)	101	(1)	95	(1)	35	(2)	63	(3)
	II	90	(2)	144	(1)	65	(1)	47	(3)		
	III					29	(3)				

TABLE 9 (Continued)

Determination	Study Period**	Patient 1	2	3	4	5
Reticuloendothelial		Hepatosplenomegaly. Bacilli in liver and lymph nodes	No bacilli in liver and lymph nodes, but giant cells & granulomas present. No hepatosplenomegaly	No hepatosplenomegaly. Bacilli present in liver and lymph nodes	No hepatosplenomegaly. Bacilli present in liver and lymph nodes	No hepatosplenomegaly. Bacilli present in liver and lymph nodes
Bones (X-ray)		normal	demineralized digits, remineralized during therapy	digits demineralized during febrile reaction	demineralized digits	demineralized digits; loss of terminal phalangeal tufts; septic arthritis of thumb

** Study Period: See corresponding footnote for Table 4.

TABLE 10

Gastrointestinal and Hepatic Function in Five Patients with Leprosy

Determination	Study Period**	Patient 1 Mean Value	Patient 1 Speci-mens	Patient 2 Mean Value	Patient 2 Speci-mens	Patient 3 Mean Value	Patient 3 Speci-mens	Patient 4 Mean Value	Patient 4 Speci-mens	Patient 5 Mean Value	Patient 5 Speci-mens
Cholesterol	I	118	(8)	199	(3)	161	(1)	184	(9)	224	(7)
(total)	II	130	(16)	228	(15)	144	(1)	185	(14)		
serum	III					145	(12)				
Cholesterol	I	34	(1)	61	(1)	45	(1)	—			
(free)	II	49	(1)	67	(1)	59	(1)	—			
plasma	III					—					
Triglycerides	I	77	(1)	41	(1)	58	(1)	—		—	
plasma	II	83	(1)	56	(1)	157	(1)	—			
	III					—					
Phospholipids	I	157	(1)	255	(1)	233	(1)	—		—	
plasma	II	175	(1)	294	(1)	292	(1)	—			
	III					—					
Thymol	I	6–7	(2)	0	(1)	0	(1)	1–11	(16)	9–12	(12)
turbidity	II	9–12	(11)	3	(10)	3	(1)	4–7	(11)		
serum	III					4	(12)				
Cephalin	I	4 plus	(2)	1	(1)	1	(1)	0–4	(13)	3–4	(4)
flocculation,	II	2 plus	(10)	0	(1)	2	(1)	2–4	(14)		
serum		4 plus									
	III					2	(10)				

TABLE 10 (Continued)

Determination	Study Period**	Patient 1 Mean Value	Patient 1 Speci-mens	Patient 2 Mean Value	Patient 2 Speci-mens	Patient 3 Mean Value	Patient 3 Speci-mens	Patient 4 Mean Value	Patient 4 Speci-mens	Patient 5 Mean Value	Patient 5 Speci-mens
Glutamic oxaloacetic transaminase serum	I	normal	(2)	normal	(1)	normal	(1)	normal	(9)	normal	(3)
	II	normal	(7)	normal	(1)	normal	(4)	normal	(3)		
	III					24 max: 71	(11)				
Glutamic pyruvic trans-aminase serum	I	normal	(2)	normal	(1)	normal	(1)	normal	(10)	normal	(3)
	II	normal	(7)	normal	(1)	—		normal	(3)		
	III					23 max: 78	(12)				
Bilirubin serum	I	normal	(2)	—		—		normal	(11)	normal	(1)
	II	normal	(6)	normal	(5)	normal	(2)	normal	(2)		
	III					normal	(13)				
Vitamin A serum	I	18	(1)			48	(1)	—		—	
	II	—		—		44	(1)	—		—	
	III					—					
Carotene serum	I	44	(1)			70	(1)	—		—	
	II	—		—		120	(1)				
	III					—					

** Study Period: See corresponding footnote for Table 4.

TABLE 11

Abnormalities in Renal Function in Five Patients with Leprosy

		Patient									
		1		2		3		4		5	
Determination	Study Period**	Mean Value	Speci-mens	Mean Value	Speci-mens	Mean Value	Speci-mens	Mean Value	Speci-mens	Mean Value	Speci-mens
Urea nitrogen,	I	normal	(1)	normal	(1)	normal	(1)	normal	(14)	normal	(7)
plasma	II	normal	(15)	normal	(1)	normal	(6)	normal	(14)		
(mg/100 ml)	III					15,max:25	(15)				
Creatinine,	I	normal	(2)	normal	(1)	normal	(1)	normal	(8)	normal	(2)
serum	II	normal	(1)	normal	(2)	normal	(1)	normal	(12)		
(mg/100 ml)	III					1.1	(9)				
						max: 1.5					
2 hr. urine	I	normal	(2)	—		normal	(1)	normal	(1)	normal	(1)
excretion of	II	—		normal	(1)	54%	(1)	—			
Phenolsulfon-	III					34%	(1)				
phthalein (%)											
Creatinine	I	normal	(1)	normal	(1)	normal	(1)	normal	(3)	normal	(9)
clearance	II	normal	(1)	—		normal	(1)	normal	(2)		
(ml/min.)	III					45	(2)				

TABLE 11 (Continued)

		Patient									
		1		2		3		4		5	
Determination	Study Period**	Mean Value	Speci-mens	Mean Value	Speci-mens	Mean Value	Speci-mens	Mean Value	Speci-mens	Mean Value	Speci-mens
Maximal urine specific gravity > 1.025	I	normal	(3)	normal	(2)	normal	(1)	normal	(1)	normal	(1)
	II	normal	(3)	normal	(1)	normal	(1)	normal	(1)	1.023	(2)
	III					1.016	(1)				
Protein, 24 hour urine, (gm)	I	0	(5)	0	(1)	—		0	(1)	0.1 max: 0.4	(4)
	II	—		0	(2)	0	(2)				
	III					0.5 max: 0.8	(14)				
Urinalysis	I	normal	(9)	normal	(4)	normal	(2)	0–2 plus protein	(19)	normal, except postop.	(9)
	II	normal	(19)	normal	(2)	normal	(7)	0–1 plus protein	(23)		
	III					WBC, 3 casts max: 30	(25)				

** Study Period: See corresponding footnote for Table 4.

TABLE 12

Urinary Corticosteroid Excretion in Five Patients with Leprosy

	Patient				
	1	2	3	4	5
Summary:	Decreased responsiveness to ACTH and SU4885. Decreased output of 17KS	Probably a decreased response to ACTH and SU4885. Decreased output of 17KS	Initially normal response to ACTH, but possible decreased response during "reaction." Decreased output of 17KS	Normal response to ACTH and SU-4885. Possibly decreased 17KS output	Normal response to ACTH and SU-4885. Probably decreased 17KS output
17 Hydroxycorticosteroids (17OHCS)	Normal = 4–14 mg/24 hours				
Number of collections	22, including 12 with ACTH & 2 with SU4885 stimulation	10, including 1 with ACTH & 2 with SU4885 stimulation	18, including 5 with ACTH & 2 with SU4885 stimulation	21, including 1 with ACTH & 2 with SU4885 stimulation	4, including 1 with ACTH & 2 with SU4885 stimulation
Mean	10.0	6.9	9.7	8.7	16.2
Range of values (mg/24 hours)	0.9–21.5	0.7–14.3	2.4–18.6	2.6–24.8	8.4–21.4

TABLE 12 (Continued)

	Patient 1	Patient 2	Patient 3	Patient 4	Patient 5
Results	6 < normal 12 = in normal range 4 > normal	2 < normal 7 = in normal range 1 > normal	2 < normal 12 = in normal range 4 > normal	5 < normal 13 = in normal range 3 > normal	1 = in normal range 3 > normal
17 Ketosteroids (17KS)	Normal = 10–24 mg/24 hours				
Number of collections	19, including 10 with ACTH & 1 with SU4885	7, including 2 with ACTH stimulation	19, including 4 with ACTH & 1 with SU4885	21, including 1 with ACTH & 2 with SU4885	4, including 1 with ACTH & 2 with SU4885
Mean	6.1	8.2	6.7	10.2	8.5
Range of values (mg/24 hrs.)	0.3–16.0	3.3–14.6	1.4–12.5	2.6–17.2	6.8–9.9
Results	15 < normal 4 = in normal range	5 < normal 2 = in normal range	16 < normal 3 = in normal range	10 < normal 11 = in normal range	4 < normal

TABLE 13

Plasma Corticoid Values*

Following ACTH Administration in Five Patients with Leprosy

Study Period **	Patient														
	1			2			3			4			5		
	Before	After	ACTH	Before	After	ACTH	Before	After	ACTH	Before	After	ACTH	Before	After	ACTH
I	22	19	25uIV	13	41	25uIV	16	46	25uIV	7	38	40uIV	12	32	25uIV
		no response			normal			normal			normal			normal	
II (early)	9	20	25uIV	14	37	50uIV	20	13	25uIV						
		not a significant increase			normal			no response							
II (late)	15	35	50uIV												
		normal													
III (early)								5	40uIM daily x7						
								no response							
III (late)							11	27	20uIV						
								increase to slightly above normal value							

* Plasma Corticoids: normal limits=5–20 μgm/100ml.

** Study Period: See corresponding footnote for Table 4.

TABLE 14
Reproductive Function
in Five Patients with Leprosy

	Patient				
	1	2	3	4	5
Seminal Emission	Seminal emission abnormal: no sperm present, volume reduced (0.5 ml), acid-fast bacilli present, and viscosity greater than normal.	Cannot produce seminal emission; no sperm in touch preparation of incised epididymis; sperm seen in one urine specimen.	Seminal emission abnormal: volume decreased (0.7 ml). 17% of sperm show abnormal morphology. Sperm count is normal (73×10^6/ml) and motility is normal. Viscosity of emission is normal.	Seminal emission normal; volume 2.8 ml, count 33.8×10^6/ml, more than 80% motile for 1 hour and more than 90% show normal morphology. No bacilli in emission.	Unable to produce seminal emission Urethral discharge following prostatic massage contains acid-fast bacilli.
Testicles	Testicles: atrophic, with many acid-fast bacilli and no sperm. Size: 4.0x2.0 cm	Testicles: partial fibrosis and atrophy with decrease in spermatogenesis. Size: 6.0x4.5 cm	Testicles: normal on examination and biopsy; no bacilli in emission or testes. Size: 4.0x3.0 cm	Testicles: inflammation and fibrosis, many acid-fast bacilli present. Size: 4.0x3.0 cm	Testicles; inflammation and fibrosis, sperm and bacilli are present. Size: 4.5x3.1 cm

TABLE 14 (Continued)

	Patient				
	1	2	3	4	5
Gonadotrophins	Gonadotrophins increased to eunuchoid range (500 mouse units)	Gonadotrophins slightly elevated (> 65 and < 240 mouse units)	Gonadotrophins normal.	Gonadotrophins normal.	
Urinary ketosteroids (17KS)	Urinary ketosteroid output decreased (range 0.3–16.0 mg/day).	Urinary ketosteroid output decreased (range 3.3–14.6 mg/day).	Urinary ketosteroid output decreased (range 1.4–12.5 mg/day).	Urinary ketosteroids show some low output days, but are usually normal 2.6–17.2 mg/day).	Urinary ketosteroids decreased (6.8–9.9 mg/day).
Marital status	Unmarried; has never had intercourse.	Unmarried, but had had intercourse weekly until illness began; for 8 months has been unable to maintain erection. Has had gonorrhea.	Unmarried, adolescent; has never had intercourse.	Unmarried; intercourse weekly; has had gonorrhea.	Married, with 2 children, separated for 4 years. Impotent since illness began 4 years ago. Has had gonorrhea. Has balanoposthitis.
Seminal vesiculogram	Normal	Partial obstruction	Normal	Partial obstruction	Partial obstruction

TABLE 15
Additional Laboratory Studies
in Five Patients with Leprosy

Determination	Patient 1	2	3	4	5
Gastric analysis	n*	n	—**	n	—
Audiogram	n	n	initially unsatisfactory, then normal	n	—
Serum electrolytes	n	n	n	n	n
Red cell osmotic fragility	n	n	n	borderline low	n
Xylose tolerance test	n	n	n	—	—
Amylase, serum	n	n	n	n	—
Bromsulfphthalein retention	n	n	n	n	2–12 (2 specimens)
Uric acid, serum	n	n	n, increasing to 4.2	—	—

* n = normal

** — = not done

TABLE 15 (Continued)

	Patient				
Determination	1	2	3	4	5
Prothrombin time	17 sec. (control: 13)	n	n	n	n
Coagulation time (siliconized tube)	n	n	normal, once; 60 min., once	n	n
Hemoglobin electrophoresis	"A" present "C,S" absent	"A" present "C,S" absent	"A" present "C,S" absent	"A" present "C,S" absent	"A" present "C,S" absent
Vitamin C, serum	n	n	n	—	—
Cerebrospinal fluid	n	n	n	n	n
Lactic dehydrogenase, serum	n	n	n	—	—
Urobilinogen,					
fecal	n	n	n	n	n
urine	n	n	n	n	n
Acid phosphatase serum	n	n	n	n	n
Magnesium, serum	n	n	n	n	n

TABLE 15 (Continued)

Determination	Patient 1	2	3	4	5
Copper, serum	n	n	n	—	—
Sex Chromatin buccal mucosa	—	—	male	—	—
Amyloid stains					
skin	neg.	neg.	neg.	neg.	neg.
kidney	neg.	neg.	neg.	neg.	neg.
liver	neg.	neg.	neg.	neg.	neg.
testicles	neg.	neg.	neg.	neg.	neg.
gum	neg.	neg.	neg.	neg.	neg.
jejunem	neg.	neg.	neg.	neg.	neg.
rectum	—	—	—	neg.	—
lymph node	neg.	neg.	neg.	neg.	neg.
prostate	neg.	neg.	neg.	neg.	neg.
bone marrow	neg.	neg.	neg.	neg.	neg.
Gerota's fat	neg.	neg.	neg.	neg.	neg.
muscle	neg.	neg.	neg.	neg.	neg.
breast	—	—	—	neg.	—
spermatic fascia	neg.	neg.	—	neg.	—

TABLE 15 (Continued)

	Patient				
Determination	1	2	3	4	5
Electrocardiogram	n	n	n	n	n
Electroenceph-alogram	n	n	n	n	n
Fasting blood sugar, plasma	n	n	n	n	n
Glucose toler-ance test	n	n	n	n	n
Alkaline phos-phatase, serum	n	n	42, decreasing to 7 during fever	n	n
Glucose 6-phos-phate dehydro-genase, serum	n	—	—	n	—
Hydroxyproline, urine	n	n	—	—	—
Bleeding time	n	n	n	n	n
Thyroid stimu-lating hormone, plasma	n	n	n	—	—

TABLE 15 (Continued)

Determination	Patient 1	2	3	4	5
Basal metabolic rate	normal once; −11.3 once	n	n	n	n
Radioactive iodine uptake	n	n	n	n	n
Red cell thyroxine I^{131} uptake	n	n	n	—	—
Thyroxine bound iodine, serum	n	n	n	—	—
Calcium, serum	n	n	n	n	n
Phosphorus, serum	n	n	n	n	n
X-ray, chest	n	n	n	n	n
X-ray, skull	n	n	n	n	n
GI series	hepatosplenomegaly	n	n	*Ascaris*	n
Barium enema	n	n	n	n	n

TABLE 15 (Continued)

Determination	Patient 1		Patient 2		Patient 3		Patient 4		Patient 5	
Bone age	n		n		n		n		n	
I.V.P.	–		–		–		n		n	
Bacteriologic cultures	Mean Value	Speci-mens	Mean Value	Speci-mens	Mean Value	Speci-mens	Mean Value	Speci-mens	Mean Value	Speci-mens
for *M. Tuberculosis*										
Biopsies	0	(10)	0	(13)	0	(9)	0	(13)	0	(2)
Body fluids & secretions	0	(14)	0	(14)	0	(10)	0*	(9)	0**	(5)
for fungi	*C. tropicalis* *Penicillium* 0	(1) (2) (12)	0	(7)	*C. albicans* 0	(3) (14)	*C. albicans* 0	(2) (15)	0	(4)

* One gastric washing specimen contained a few colonies of *scotochromogen*, Runyon II.
** Tuberculosis developed subsequently (1965), proved by sputum culture, and responded to INH and PAS therapy.

TABLE 15 (Continued)

Bacteriologic cultures for common pathogens	Patient 1	2	3	4	5
Ulcerations	*β-streptococcus*	—	—	—	—
Sputum	0	*S. aureus* (hemolytic)	0	0	0
Throat	0	0	0	*β-streptococcus*	0
Urine	*Klebsiella*	0	*β-streptococcus*	0	*S. aureus* (hemolytic)
Wound	0	—	*S. aureus* (hemolytic)	—	*S. aureus* (hemolytic)
Intestinal parasites	*H. nana*	*H. nana* *T. trichiura*	*H. nana* *E. histolytica*	*H. nana* *A. lumbricoides* *T. trichiura* *G. lamblia*	*A. lumbricoides* *T. trichiura* *N. americanus*

TABLE 16
Febrile Reactions in Patient 4
Alterations Observed

	Jan.	Feb. – March	April	May
Temperature increase	8°C.	3°C.	7°C.	7°C.
Weight decrease	2.0 kg	2.5 kg	3.0 kg	3.5 kg
ESR increase	70	76	80	40
Hematocrit decrease	13	5	11	12
Reticulocytes increase	2.3	2.2	2.3	4.0

GLOSSARY

DDS. Dapsone or Avlosulfon® Ayerst. The structure is shown in a footnote in the Methods section.

DPT. Thiocarbanilide, or CIBA 1906. The structure is shown in a footnote in the Methods section.

B-663. An experimental antileprosy drug, derived from rimizine dye. The structure is shown in a footnote in the Methods section.

DIMORPHOUS ("BORDERLINE") LEPROSY. A reactive form of leprosy in which characteristics of both lepromatous and tuberculoid leprosy occur. The lepromin test may be positive or negative, and bacillary proliferation and granulomatous reactions are observed.

GLOBUS (PLEURAL: GLOBI). A mass of adherent leprosy bacilli, believed by many to be within the remnants of a phagocytic macrophage. When masses of bacilli are seen in cells with preserved membranes and nuclei, the cells are called "lepra cells," "foam cells" or "Virchow's cells," terms which are commonly used interchangeably.

INDETERMINATE LEPROSY. An early or uncharacteristic stage of leprosy in which bacillary-positive skin macules occur. The patients are clinically well in this stage, and later progress to either the lepromatous or tuberculoid type. The lepromin test may be positive or negative.

LEPROMATOUS LEPROSY. The progressive disease in which the patient exhibits minimal resistance to growth and dissemination of leprosy bacilli. Bacilli occur in large numbers in skin and mucous membranes. The lepromin skin test is negative. Until the disease is arrested, the patients are infective. They frequently develop complications, such as tuberculosis and amyloidosis, which shorten life expectancy.

LEPROMIN. A sterile suspension of emulsified lepromas (nodules from leprosy patients), used for intradermal skin testing in leprosy since its original description by Mitsuda. No reaction occurs in lepromatous patients. Normal individuals and tuberculoid patients usually exhibit a granulomatous nodule at 48 hours and at 21 days. The reaction in dimorphous and indeterminate leprosy is variable.

LEPROSY. The chronic infectious disease caused by *Mycobacterium leprae,* an acid-fast bacillus similar in appearance to the causative organism of tuberculosis. *M. leprae* is different from *M. tuberculosis* in that it predominantly attacks skin and peripheral nerves, sparing the lungs and central nervous system. Both organisms may be found in the reticuloendothelial system, and tuberculosis is not uncommon in patients with leprosy. Unlike the tubercle bacillus, *M. leprae* cannot be cultivated in vitro on artificial media, and does not ordinarily cause progressive disseminated disease when inoculated into other species. Several types of leprosy are recognized. Among these are lepromatous, tuberculoid, indeterminate, and dimorphous or "borderline." Other classifications emphasize anatomical features such as: diffuse, nodular, neural, reactional, or maculoanesthetic.

MURINE LEPROSY. The disease of rodents caused by *Mycobacterium leprae murium*, an organism similar but not identical to the human leprosy bacillus, *M. leprae*.

STAIN. Mycobacteria resist decolorization with mineral acids after staining with aniline dyes. This property is utilized in the Ziehl-Nielsen stain (for tissue emulsions and other fluid suspensions of bacteria), and in the Fite stain of paraffin-embedded tissue sections.

STUDY PERIOD I. The period of observation and nonspecific treatment prior to institution of specific antileprosy chemotherapy. The length of this period varied from two to three and one-half months:

Patient 1	2 mos.
Patient 2	2 mos.
Patient 3	2 mos.
Patient 4	3½ mos.
Patient 5	3 mos.

STUDY PERIOD II. The period of administration of specific chemotherapy, while observations continued. This period varied from three to five months.

		Drugs used
Patient 1	5 mos.	DDS
Patient 2	5 mos.	DDS
Patient 3	3 mos.	DDS
Patient 4	3 mos.	DDS + B-663

The treatment of patient 5 began after the studies described in this monograph were completed.

STUDY PERIOD III. A reactional period in patient 3, lasting four months, during which prednisone was administered intermittently and antileprosy chemotherapy was changed from DDS to DPT.

TUBERCULOID LEPROSY. A form of leprosy characterized by a high resistance to the propagation of leprosy bacilli. The disease is usually self-limited.

REFERENCES

Arnold, H. L. 1966. Paradoxes and misconceptions in leprosy. *J. Am. Med. Assoc.* 196:647–50.

Aycock, W. L., and Gordon, J. E. 1947. Leprosy in veterans of American wars. *Am. J. Med. Sci.* 214:329.

Beddow, R. M., and Tilden, I. L. 1960. Malabsorption syndrome due to amyloidosis of the intestine secondary to lepromatous leprosy. Report of a case. *Ann. Int. Med.* 53:1017.

Binford, C. 1958. Leprosy as a diagnostic problem in surgical pathology. *So. Med. J., J. So. Med. Assoc.* 51:200.

Black, S. H. 1938. The pathology of leprosy. *Am. Assoc. Advanc. Sci. Symposium* 1:97.

Blumberg, B. S.; Melartin, L.; Lechat, M., and Guinto, R. S. 1967. Association between lepromatous leprosy and Australia antigen. *Lancet* 2:173.

Bonar, B. E., and Rabson, A. S. 1957. Gynecologic aspects of leprosy. *Obstet. and Gyn.* 9:33.

Browne, S. G., and Hogerzeil, L. M. 1962. "B663" in the treatment of leprosy. Preliminary report of a pilot trial. *Lep. Rev.* 33:6.

Bullock, W. E. 1968. Studies of immune mechanisms in leprosy. I. Depression of delayed allergic response to skin test antigens. *N.E.J.M.* 278:298.

Burgess, P. 1951. *Born of Those Years.* New York: Henry Holt.

———. 1940. *Who Walk Alone.* New York: Holt, Rinehart & Winston.

Canizares, O.; Costello, M.; and Gigli, I. 1962. Erythema nodosum type of lepra reaction. *Arch. Derm.* 85:29.

Cathcart, E. S., et al. 1961. The relationship of the latex fixation test to the clinical and serologic manifestations of leprosy. *Am. J. Med.* 31:758.

Cochrane, R. G. 1962. Chemotherapy of leprosy. *The Practitioner* 188:67.

———. 1959. *Leprosy in Theory and Practice.* Bristol: John Wright. See especially: technique of skin scrapings, p. 369.

Davey, T. F., and Currie, G. 1956. Clinical trial of diphenyl thiourea Compound SU 1906 (CIBA 15095E) in the treatment of leprosy. Progress during the first year. *Lep. Rev.* 27:94.

Derbes, V. J., et al. 1961. The Lucio form of diffuse leprosy. Case in a Louisiana Negro. *Int. J. Lep.* 29(2): 200–215.

Dogliotti, M., and Fazio, M. 1960. Biopsy of the liver in lepromatous leprosy. *Acta Hepatospl.* 7:7–24.

Doull, J. A. 1954. Leprosy. *Vet. Admin. Tech. Bull.* TB-10-98. Washington, D.C.: Gov. Printing Office.

———. 1963. "Chairman's Closing Remarks," in *The Pathogenesis of Leprosy,* ed. G. E. W. Wolstenholme. Boston: Little, Brown. pp. 97–99.

———; Guinto, R. S.; and Mabalay, M. C. 1957. Effect of BCG vaccination, lepromin testing and natural causes in inducing reactivity to lepromin and to tuberculin. *Int. J. Lep.* 25:13–37.

———; ———; and ———. 1959. The origin of natural reactivity to lepromin. The association between the Mitsuda reaction and reactions to graded doses of tuberculin. *Int. J. Lep.* 27:31–42.

———, et al. 1961. Clinical evaluation studies in lepromatous leprosy. Fourth series: 4, butoxy-4'demethylaminodiphenyl thiourea (DPT), amodiaquin, and 4-4' diaminodiphenyl sulfone (DDS) 2.5 mg and 4 mgm per kg of body weight. *Int. J. Lep.* 29:291–317.

Faget, G. H. et al. 1943. The promin treatment of leprosy. *Public Health Rep.* 58:1729.

Farrow, J. 1954. *Damien the Leper.* Garden City: Doubleday. (1st ed. 1937, Sheed and Ward.)

Fernandez, J. M. M. 1940. The early reaction induced by lepromin. *Int. J. Lep.* 8:1–14.

Fite, G. L. 1943. Leprosy from the histologic point of view. *Arch. Path.* 35:611–44.

———; Cambre, P. J.; and Turner, M. H. 1947. Procedure for demonstrating lepra bacilli in paraffin sections. *Arch. Path.* 43:624–25.

Goodwin, C. S. 1968. Antipyretic and anti-inflammatory action of flufenamic acid in acute reaction of lepromatous leprosy. *Lancet.* 2:854–55.

Grabstald, H., and Swan, L. L. 1951. Genitourinary lesions in leprosy. With special reference to the problem of atrophy of the testes. *J. Am. Med. Assoc.* 149:1287–91.

Gray, H. H., and Dreisback, J. A. 1961. Leprosy among foreign missionaries in northern Nigeria. *Int. J. Lep.* 29:279–290.

Greene, Graham. 1961. *A Burnt-Out Case.* New York: Viking.

Guinto, R. S.; Mabalay, M. C.; and Doull, J. A. 1962. Cutaneous responses to lepromin and to other mycobacterial antigens (human, avian and Battey tuberculins and human and avian tubercle bacilli). *Int. J. Lep.* 30:152–165.

———, and ———. 1962. A note on the tuberculin reaction in leprosy. *Int. J. Lep.* 30:278–283.

Hansen, G. H. A. 1874. Indberetning til det Norske mediciniske Selskab i Christiania om en med understøttelse af selskabet foretagen reise for at anstille undersøgelser angående spedalskhedens årsager, tildels undførte sammen med forstander Hartwig. Christiania: Det Steenske Bogiykkeri. *Norsk Mag. f. Laegevidensk,* Christiania. 3R, 4, 9 Hefte, 1–88.

Hippocrates. Translated by Adams, F. 1886. *The Genuine Works of Hippocrates. Translated from the Greek with a Preliminary Discourse and Annotations, Vol. 1.* (2 vols.) New York: William Wood. p. 224.

Hutchinson, J. 1906. *On Leprosy and Fish-Eating.* London: Archibald Constable.

James, D. G., and Jopling, W. H. 1961. Sarcoidosis and leprosy. *J. Trop. Med. Hyg.* 64:42–46.

Jamison, D. G., and Vollum, R. L. 1968. Tuberculin conversion in leprous families in northern Nigeria. *Lancet.* 2:1271–72.

Job, C. K. 1961. Gynecomastia and leprous orchitis. A preliminary study. *Int. J. Lep.* 29:423–441.

Kean, B. H., and Childress, M. E. 1942. A summary of 103 autopsies on leprosy patients on the Isthmus of Panama. *Int. J. Lep.* 10:51–59.

Kher, M., and Grover, S. 1969. Glucose-6-phosphate dehydrogenase deficiency in leprosy. Letter. *Lancet* 1:1318–19.

Koch, R. 1882. Cited in Bulloch, William, *The History of Bacteriology*. London: Oxford University Press. 1960. p. 377.

Larkey, S. V. 1961. Leprosy in medieval romance: a note on Robert Henryson's "Testament of Cresseid." *Bull. Hist. Med.* 35:77–80.

Latapi, F., and Zamora, A. C. 1948. The "spotted" leprosy of Lucio (la lepra "manchada" de Lucio). An introduction to its clinical and histological study. *Int. J. Lep.* 16:421–29.

Lechat, M. F. 1962. Bone lesions in leprosy. *Int. J. Lep.* 30:125–137.

Levine, M. 1951. Hemagglutination of tuberculin sensitized sheep cells in Hansen's disease (Leprosy). *Proc. Soc. Exp. Biol. Med.* 76:171–173.

Lewis, N. G.; Fite, G. L.; and Bogen, E. 1961. Comparison of reactions to human and avian tuberculins in leprosy patients. *Int. J. Lep.* 29:355–58.

Lewis, O. 1964. Pedro Martinez: *A Mexican Peasant and his Family*. New York: Random House.

McFadzean, J. A. 1961. An investigation of the possible role of mosquitoes and bed bugs in the transmission of leprosy. *Tr. Roy. Soc. Trop. Med. Hyg.* 55:232–34.

Mabalay, M. C.; Helwig, E. B.; Tolentino, J. G.; and Binford, C. H. 1965. The histopathology and histochemistry of erythema nodosum leprosum. *Int. J. Lep.* 33:28–49.

Madrid Congress. 1953. Report of Classification Committee. *Memoria del VI Congreso Internacional de Leprologia*, p. 75.

Martin, B. 1950. *Miracle at Carville*. Garden City: Doubleday.

———. 1959. *No One must Ever Know*. Garden City: Doubleday.

Martin, F. I. R., et al. 1968. Leprous endocrinopathy. *Lancet* 2:1320–21.

Medina, R. M. 1944. Cited by Latapi, F., op. cit. 1948.

Mitsuda, K. 1919. Cited by Doull, J. A., op. cit. 1954.

———, and Ogawa, M. 1937. A study of one hundred and fifty autopsies on cases of leprosy. *Int. J. Lep.* 5:53–60.

———, 1952. *Atlas of Leprosy*. Okayama, Japan: Chotokai Foundation.

Morris, J. A., et al. 1961. Fluorescent antibody study of the human leprosy bacillus. *Bact. Proc.* 14:123.

Muelling, R. J.; Goetz, C.; and Sister H. Ross. 1960. Serum protein patterns in leprosy. Carville Survey I. *Int. J. Lep.* 28:144–154.

New York Academy of Sciences. 1966. Leprosy: twelve million victims. *The Sciences* 6:1–5.

Osler, W. 1898. Leprosy in the United States, with the report of a case. *Johns Hopkins Hosp. Bull.* No. 84.

Powell, C. S., and Swan, L. L. 1955. Leprosy: pathologic changes observed in fifty consecutive necropsies. *Am. J. Path.* 31:1131–47.

Rees, R. J. W., et al. 1967. Experimental lepromatous leprosy. *Nature* 215:599–602.

———, and Waters, M. F. 1963. The *Pathogenesis of Leprosy,* ed. G. E. W. Wolstenholem, pp. 39–55. Boston: Little, Brown.

Rogers, J. H. 1960. Coronary thrombosis, cerebral vascular accident and pulmonary embolism in leprosy. *Ann. Int. Med.* 53:746–753.

Rokstad, I. 1964. Gerhard Heinrich Armauer Hansen. *Int. J. Lep.* 32:64–70.

Saul, A., and Hill, G. J. 1963. Algunas investigaciones recientes en lepra. Communicacion preliminar de un estudio cooperative en tres casos clinicos. *Dermatologica Revista Mexicana.* 7:97–113.

Shepard, C. C. 1960. Acid-fast bacilli in nasal excretions in leprosy, and results of inoculation of mice. *Am. J. Hyg.* 71:147–57.

———. 1960. The experimental disease that follows the injection of human leprosy bacilli into foot-pads of mice. *J. Exp. Med.* 112:445–55.

———, and Kirsh, D. 1961. Fluorescent antibody stainability and other consequences of the disruption of mycobacteria. *Proc. Soc. Exp. Biol. Med.* 106:685–691.

Stevenson, R. L. 1923. *The Complete Poems of Robert Louis Stevenson.* New York: Charles Scribners. "To Mother Maryanne," on Molokai Island. p. 172.

Turk, J. L., and Water, M. F. R. 1968. Immunological basis for depression of cellular immunity and the delayed allergic response in patients with lepromatous leprosy. *Lancet* 2:436–38.

Virchow, R. 1864–65. *Die Krankhaften Geschwülste, Vol. 2.* Berlin: August Hirschwald. pp. 494–554: leprosy discussed, incl. historical refs., 6 illus., description of characteristic lepra cell; p. 514: line drawing of cell; pp. 514–515: this description translated by Fite, op. cit. 1943.

Wade, H. W., and Rodriguiez, J. N. 1940. Borderline tuberculoid leprosy. *Int. J. Lep.* 8:307.

———, 1957. A modification of the Fite formaldehyde (Fite I) method for staining acid-fast bacilli in paraffin sections. *Stain Tech.* 32:287–292.

Waldorf, D. S. et al. 1966. Impaired delayed hypersensitivity in patients with lepromatous leprosy. *Lancet* 2:773–76.

Wemambu, S. N. C., et al. 1969. Erythema Nodosum leprosum: a clinical manifestation of the Arthus phenomenon. *Lancet* 2:933–35.

Weymouth, A. 1938. *Through the Leper-Squint.* London: Selwyn & Blount.

Williams, T. W., Jr., et al. 1965. Leprosy research at the National Institutes of Health: experience with B.663 in the treatment of leprosy. *Proc.* LWM-AFIP Conf. *Int. J. Lep.* 33:3, Pt. 2, 767–775.

Wolstenholme, G. E. W. 1963. *The Pathogenesis of Leprosy.* Boston: Little, Brown.

World Health Organization. 1961. Scientific meeting on rehabilitation in leprosy. Geneva: World Health Organization.

INDEX